Dr. Kellyann's Bone Broth Breakthrough

ALSO BY DR. KELLYANN PETRUCCI

Dr. Kellyann's Bone Broth Diet

Dr. Kellyann's Bone Broth Cookbook

The 10-Day Belly Slimdown

Dr. Kellyann's Cleanse and Reset

Dr. Kellyann's

Bone Broth Breakthrough

Turn Back the Clock.

Reset Your Scale.

Replenish Your Power.

Kellyann Petrucci, MS, ND

RODALE.
NEW YORK

Published in the United States by Rodale Books, an imprint of Random House, a division of Penguin Random House LLC, New York.
RodaleBooks.com
RandomHouseBooks.com

Rodale Books is a registered trademark, and the Circle colophon is a trademark of Penguin Random House LLC.

Library of Congress Cataloging-in-Publication Data is available upon request.

ISBN 978-0-593-57912-1
Ebook ISBN 978-0-593-57913-8

Printed in the United States of America

Book design by Andrea Lau
Jacket design by Anna Bauer Carr
Jacket photograph by Keith Major

10 9 8 7 6 5 4 3 2 1

First Edition

To my Momma:
Thank you for inspiring me to always grow,
To be sweet, level, and loyal,
To deflect anger and keep love in my heart,
To be open and creative.

To my Poppa:
Thank you for inspiring me to live with integrity,
To transform myself and others,
To be a positive force,
To always see possibilities and be savage in pursuing them.

Thank you both for your struggle and hard work,
For holiday talent shows and years (decades!) of dance lessons,
For encouraging me to go and figure out my own jam,
For always making sure I knew I was loved.

The further I go in my life,
the more grateful I am
for that unshakeable foundation.

Contents

Introduction

I t's been nearly twenty years since I froze time. I know it sounds crazy, but it's true. If you're wondering if I mean that in a deal-with-the-devil way, that's not it. I made a deal with my cells. I found a way to tune in and give them what they needed, and in return my skin stopped aging. I stopped putting on weight. And I had more energy for everything I wanted to do with my life. I've continued to honor my end of that bargain all these years, and my strategies haven't failed me.

I know the time-freezing thing is real because every day I'm mistaken for being younger than I am—often by a decade, frequently by two. The other day I texted the cover photo for this book to a colleague, and the response I got was, *Wow you're a freak of nature.* I'm not gonna lie: It feels good to look good, feel strong, and be confident. It feels good to be free of *worry* about aging, too. Because the secret I unlocked brought magic to my life that transcends any scale or clothing size, or even the birth date on my driver's license.

But the best part for me really comes down to you. My entire career has been about helping people transform—even before I figured out how to do that for myself. For me, it's the most rewarding work in the world. I wake up every morning eager to share my methods, secrets, and encouragement with somebody new. Or with anybody that needs a boost. My friends joke that if you hang around me long enough, you inevitably start to look better. It sounds ridiculous, but it's pretty accurate. If I know you, I sprinkle you with nutrition and lifestyle recommendations—and in all likelihood bring a little extra health, vitality, and beauty into your life. That's what I set out to do in designing a lifestyle that has worked for me for almost two decades—one that I know can work for you, too.

I want you to imagine yourself ten years from now, or twenty, or more. And I want you to picture Future You looking amazing. Ageless. Not a day older than you look today. Now imagine that beauty and vitality coming from inside you, like a light. That's the challenge. That's what we're working on: giving you a future of beauty and health that emanates from the inside out. It's a beauty that won't wash away with your makeup or crumple when the Spanx come off.

I know it can seem impossible, especially when you find yourself moving through this world like you and your body aren't in sync—or worse, like you're trying to be invisible. If that's where you are today, I want to assure you there's a way to get your confidence back and get on a path toward hope, health, and gorgeousness. You *can* have a bone broth breakthrough of your own.

If you're thinking the word "breakthrough" is a bold claim (especially when combined with a soup!), here's why I chose it: I wanted a word that implies something substantial and important. I had busting-out-of-a-cocoon level change in mind, because that's what this journey has been for me and for the hundreds of thousands of other people who've gone on it with me.

When I began exploring and recommending bone broth years ago, I thought, *THIS is my big discovery*. My lightning in a bottle. My purpose in life. And I ran with that for a long time because bone broth continually changes physical health in ways that amaze me.

But through the years, as I've curated success stories in my own life and in everyone who has let me be their guide, I've discovered that the transformations kicked off by the bone broth lifestyle go beyond weight loss, beyond great skin—even beyond anything strictly physical.

Do you remember the game Mouse Trap? It was one of our first lessons in cause and effect as children. Every action triggered another piece to fall. I see bone broth as that first action, the trigger piece, in resetting health and stopping aging. The cascade of effects that follows get bigger and better over time.

If you're wondering why this all matters so much to me, remember that my focus is different from most doctors or dietitians you've listened to before. I'm a board-certified naturopathic doctor. By definition that means I help people establish optimal health by guiding their bodies *back to the way they're supposed to work*. Rather than just suppressing symptoms by handing out pills or standard diet plans, naturopathic doctors work to identify the underlying causes of health struggles like excess weight, fatigue, and aging skin.

I'm telling you about the kind of work I do because I want you to know and trust that I'm the best-qualified person to help you make a deal with your own cells to turn back time, reset your scale, and replenish your power. Let's get started!

PART ONE

The Breakthrough

f you've read any of my previous books or know me from social media or television, you may know that most of my work focuses on specific Bone Broth Diets over periods of 1, 3, 5, 10, and 21 days. I designed each of those plans to help you kick off a new phase of health and wellness—and each as a system you can return to anytime you want to cleanse and reset your body. The logical next question that I get all the time is, *What's next? How do I return to my after-diet life without backsliding?* This book is the answer.

Another question I frequently hear comes from people who choose not to diet—who don't want to live with the short-term restrictions dieting implies. They want to know, *How can I feel and look fantastic by making changes I can live with long term?* Maybe this is you, sharing those goals of optimal weight, a healthy gut, glowing skin, and a thriving immune system—but wanting to get there through steady lifestyle adjustments rather than a more strict plan that's meant to bring change within a temporary time frame. This book is the answer for that, too.

Or maybe you're at square one, sick of feeling heavy or sluggish or depleted, ready to make a change, curious about the healing powers of bone broth but unsure where to start. If so, you can get on the right track with these pages.

No matter what brings you here, I get it. It's hard figuring out how to center and strengthen yourself and bring out your glow. It's especially hard while taking care of work and home, along with spouses and kids and parents and friends and pets and . . . who am I missing? Oh yeah, taking care of *you*.

Wherever your starting point might be, I'm excited to bring you this book that goes deeper than diet—because I want us to talk about how you can be lean and strong, and energized and flourishing for the long haul. I am going to empower you to tune into what your body needs and to demand that those needs are satisfied. I'm going to show you how to design your own perfect meal plan, how to fit activity you can do joyfully into your schedule, how to power down and recharge, and how to embrace what I call "stamina-care." I am also going to introduce you to a term called "slim-gestion," which embodies the truth that the power to lose weight lies with first healing your gut.

The question is, Where do we start?

Whether you feel like you need a total health overhaul or just subtle change, it's probably because extra pounds, sleepless nights, and unacceptable stressors have been accumulating, like dust bunnies under the couch, for years. It didn't happen overnight.

Turning it around won't happen instantly either. I like to say that the only instant thing in my life is a pot. That's why I was very strategic in laying out this book in three parts for you, with a foundation in Part One, a structure in Part Two, and a manual of suggestions and solutions for some of the most common problems women encounter in Part Three, which comes complete with dozens of delicious, healing recipes. And, of course, throughout the whole book, I'll teach you everything you need to know about bone broth while showing you how adding it to your daily diet is the single greatest thing you can do to kick-start your new lifestyle and foster glowing health and longevity.

Here in Part One, it's time to talk about mindset—the bedrock of every success. If you've picked up this book, it means you're committed to making changes, and that may be the single biggest step. But as you move forward, you've got to be mentally prepared to embrace change, to prioritize good health (and the beauty that comes with it!), and to set a course that won't be deterred when you inevitably encounter resistance.

With that in mind, let's talk about the energy, beauty, and power that are uniquely yours, and about how you can nurture those best parts of yourself to turn back the clock, reset the scale, and replenish your power. It's time to get your breakthrough started!

Chapter 1

What's That Magic?

W hat's that special magic that some women have?
You know the ones I'm talking about. They have a magnetism that draws people to them. Even when it seems like everybody else is battling bloat, constipation, thinning hair, crepe-y skin, and belly fat, they look and feel amazing. Theirs is an ethereal beauty that transcends weight, height, or age.

When you see someone walking through the world with this kind of beauty and energy, you want to know more about her, to get closer. You want to talk and laugh with her. You want to know about her workout, her makeup, her hairdresser, her posture, her life. And you want to know what the heck she eats. I mean, is this an edamame-only situation? Or does she only eat before noon? What is the combination of nutrients nourishing her to this totally boss life? Like bystanders from the diner scene in *When Harry Met Sally*, you're thinking, *I'll have what she's having,* because she is flourishing.

Women like this are beautiful, but what they're all about runs even deeper. Their attitude, confidence, fitness, humor, strength—it's all a part of that "it factor."

Years ago when I was living in London, I would pop on the Eurostar for a quick train ride to France. I loved it there because I was so enthralled with the sexy culture. I kept hearing a French saying: "je ne sais quoi." Technically it translates to, "I don't know what," but it's used to describe an indefinable, attractive, extraordinary characteristic (as in, "She had an irresistible je ne sais quoi").

The woman with je ne sais quoi walks down the street and feels light on her feet, at peace with who she is. She radiates positive energy. Her eyes sparkle. You know whatever is happening on the inside must be good because, on the outside, she's magnetic. I fell in love with this idea—and I became desperate to help my patients find it. Yes, I wanted them to reach a healthy weight and get their biometrics in order, but after we achieved that, I wanted more for them. I wanted them to have je ne sais quoi.

I always want you to take your health journey one step further. When I say I believe you can have it all, that's not lip service. And I've seen it enough times to know you can do it. This is a touchstone in both my personal and professional life. When I'm helping a patient achieve a transformation, there are all the deliberate steps we take to reach a goal, and then there's that moment when the je ne sais quoi comes into play. You start moving through the world with a little more ease and confidence—and then, *there* it is, just as surely as if you'd flipped a switch.

Hard to believe it was a humble, ancient food that helped me get to this place in my life and bring so many amazing people through their own transformations, but that's exactly what happened. Reading about, cooking, sipping, and sharing the benefits of bone broth were all changes that opened me up little by little to a new lifestyle—one that makes me feel refreshed, attractive, and strong.

This is the concept that inspired me to write these pages, to dig into what happened to me—what has happened to thousands of patients and readers who've had breakthroughs like mine. I did it because I know full well that the "it factor" women we admire have doesn't just happen on Day 21 or 30 of a diet or fitness plan. In fact, that's when it's *just beginning*. That's when the momentum of those first successes starts trending toward a version of her who doesn't just tentatively look better and feel better. She *is* better. The changes are obvious on the outside—but they're also soul deep.

That kind of breakthrough, built on the small act of adding one nourishing, replenishing thing to your life to kick off that cascade of good things, is what I want for you. I believe you can achieve it and maintain it. And I'm here to walk you through the growth and changes that will make it possible.

Are You Interrupted?

True confession: I'm a closet profiler. Call it a gift or call it a curse, but if I'm meeting you, talking with you, or even watching you walk down the street, chances are I'm trying to understand your mood, your story, and your energy. My intentions, I promise, are good. After more than two decades of guiding people through health and beauty transformations, I've learned to embrace this habit that helps me triage new patients and clients.

In other words, I see you. When I see a woman who's walking on air, I want to jump up and down for her, ask questions, and take notes. When I see someone who's obviously feeling low, I wonder what's dragging her down and what it would take to lift her up.

I know there's a way, because I see some of the most extreme cases imaginable:

- Women who are 50, 80, or even 100 pounds overweight
- Women who are so addicted to sugar that it comprises the bulk of their diets

- Women stuck in self-defeating patterns of overexercising, overeating, and overstressing
- Women who put themselves last for so long that they become neglected in every way—their health, their diet, their happiness, and their sense of self-love
- Women who are waking up as empty nesters, nearing retirement and not sure how to spend the second half of their lives
- Women who still aren't sure who they are or what they want

These are women whose best lives have been *interrupted*, and it's my job to show them that if they give their bodies the right raw materials, they are going to perk up. They are going to feel better. That's why when a woman approaches me for help, I feel confident, hopeful, and happy. I *know* she's going to gain ground. I know because I see it every day, and I know because I've been an interrupted woman myself. I found a way to turn back the clock on my aging, on my weight gain, and on negative feelings that were dragging me down.

Strange but true that my entire turnaround started with a single superfood—one that's turned into an entire health movement and food category.

Bone Broth Beginnings

I'm often asked if I invented bone broth. I definitely didn't because it's been around in some form for thousands of years. But as a doctor who is utterly fascinated with the history of human nutrition (high five to all my fellow science geeks!), I kept finding references to soups and stocks, broths, and even meat-based "teas"—all with the common element of long-simmered bones and cartilage. These references were across continents, cultures, and centuries: long life soup in China, pho in Vietnam, brodo in Italy, cow foot soup in the Caribbean. There's even a soup attributed to Hippocrates, father of modern medicine. These dishes were (and still are) largely synonymous with nourishment and healing, with soothing, and sometimes even with survival. In these many forms, bone broth is an ancient food born of ancient wisdom.

It's fair to say I got a little bit obsessed about this. In truth, I still am. Maybe it was because I was at a crossroads in my own life. I was achieving professional success, but the happiness I thought would come with my accomplishments was missing. Instead I felt stressed. I was tired. And I was aging at warp speed, watching the hollows deepening under my eyes, the wrinkles in my neck getting more prominent, and my hair thinning. Alongside those physical changes, I could almost feel the spark that's always been an elemental part of what makes me dynamic waning.

For a while I played the blame game. I blamed my fatigue on my busy life as a working mom and celebrity nutritionist with a busy clinical practice. I blamed my belly fat on my pregnancies. I blamed my wrinkles and sagging skin on my years of sun exposure. I blamed my inability to lose weight on my aging metabolism. All the while, like so many patients who have come to me for help—often as their last resort—I could feel my momentum going the wrong way. I felt like the clock was ticking to make a change.

So in 2012, with kids to raise, a practice to run, bills to pay, chapters to write, and my body confidence in free fall, I followed the thread of logic I was beginning to form around bone broth as a big idea. I started simmering bones in water on the back burner of my stove. I tinkered with times and temperatures, and with adding herbs and vegetables. I stirred and tasted and seasoned. And then I lined up Mason jars on my kitchen counter and filled them with the *liquid hope* I'd been brewing.

Of course, the real test came when I started drinking the stuff. As a physician and a nutritionist—and as someone who'd studied women's dietary habits for two decades—I knew a lot about putting together a diet plan, about making sure my body is nourished. But my early experience with bone broth was in a different league from anything else I'd ever experienced. By the third week of sipping my homemade elixir every day, I was floored by what was happening in my body.

I stopped feeling thirsty all the time. I stopped having pain in my gut. I started sleeping—the kind of deep, rejuvenating sleep I hadn't experienced in years. Those dark circles under my eyes slowly started to fade. My skin became softer and more toned. My body weight started to drop and to shift, until I looked in the mirror one day and saw the kind of lean, strong dancer's body I'd had in my youth. I was in my forties. I'd never dared to expect a change like that. I didn't yet know about the miraculous powers of glycine—the bone broth component that was helping me hold on to muscle tissue while losing fat.

What I did know was that I had reclaimed the spark I'd been missing. I was practically glowing with it.

As a child, did you ever play outside for hours on a summer day, getting dirty, soaking up too much sun, and forgetting to even stop for lunch? When you finally went inside, when you gulped down that giant glass of water or lemonade, do you remember how utterly satisfied you felt? Like it was the best thing you ever tasted, and it was putting you right again? When I look back on my initial experience with adding bone broth to my routine, that's what I think of—satisfying something I'd been ignoring, even though my body was practically screaming, *For crying out loud, you're not getting what you need!*

Week after week, I was stunned by the transformation I was undergoing—even though transformation was the skill I'd been learning and honing for my entire adult life. I'd built my professional reputation on being a "body whisperer"—a doc who could guide even tough cases into great shape.

The most amazing piece of my own bone broth experience is that it didn't stop with my diet or even with my body. Momentum breeds momentum, and the cascade of positive changes taking place in the way I looked and felt quickly spilled over into my confidence, my attitude, and that je ne sais quoi that had nearly faded away. Three months after beginning to drink bone broth every day, I was *back*—fighting fit and vibrant. I couldn't wait to share my experience and the science behind it with my patients, with my friends and family—with anybody who'd listen.

In the years since that first experiment with bone broth in my own diet, I've seen that where-has-this-been-all-my-life realization play out for hundreds of thousands of other people. They stop me on the street, write emails, share their bone broth recipes, and show me before-and-after photos. I've watched the transformation of athletes, actors, dancers, mothers, grandmothers, and some of the most beautiful women in the world. Each had this "aha" experience of feeling better and looking better—and using those positive changes to create an upward spiral in their lives. Many of them want to talk about it.

I share my story because it's important to me that you know I walk this walk. I want you to understand why I am so industrious about getting bone broth into my own body every day and why I eagerly, gratefully live the lifestyle I'm going to lay out in the chapters to come. There's a world of nutrition, wellness, and beauty products out there, and I have plenty of favorites (more on those to come!), but bone broth made my own breakthrough possible. It replenished my body, renewed my appearance, and helped me recover my swagger and confidence. Along the way, it became something more to me than food or even medicine. It became the tool I most associate with healing and wellness and opening myself up to good things.

As I started recommending the food that was transforming me to my patients, I remember thinking, *How ironic that something this old, a food that's come and gone from fashion in different forms and cultures throughout history, is the cornerstone of a lifestyle that's making me feel new again.* I am a modern woman implementing an ancient remedy, and it is empowering me to reject all kinds of assumptions—about how I should look, how I should feel, when I should decide I've accomplished enough in my profession, and even when I should hang up my sexuality in favor of being over the hill.

The fact is, for as long as I've been in naturopathic medicine, my highest goal has been to nurture enough confidence for you to know that *you've got this.* Even if your life is hard right now—especially if your life is hard right now—I want to give you motivation to start with one small thing, like I did. Because this one thing can be your saving grace, too.

Nothing makes me happier than hearing from a patient, a reader, or a customer that they feel enlightened or that my advice has given them a sense of control over their diet and wellness—sometimes for the very first time. My goal in these pages is simple: I want to get you feeling great about your health, your looks, and the speed at which you are aging. I want to help you get your body working in harmony. And I want to see you take that next step—beyond the cleanse and the diet—into living this lifestyle and loving it.

And of course, we're going to do it all with a mug of liquid gold in hand. Bone broth is *the* essential tool for burning fat, reducing inflammation, harmonizing your body's digestive function, and feeding a healthy gut.

You Are the Matrix

We live in a culture that makes it all too easy to think of the body in robotic terms—like the Terminator. From that perspective, people are made up of "parts" that eventually wear out. Illness happens solely because of bad genes or unfortunate exposure to viruses or bacteria. Drugs and surgery are how we return the body to balance. This line of thinking has its logic, and its simplicity is appealing, but please, don't buy into this view of who you are and what you can do. It's fatalistic and suggests you get what you get genetically, and that's that. It's the reason I meet so many people who've resigned themselves to being overweight like their moms, or destined to develop diabetes like their dads, or even accepting of high blood pressure or heart ailments because these conditions "run in the family."

Hear this: Having the genetic possibility of developing something and developing it are miles apart. Each of us comes into this world hard-wired with some twenty thousand genes. But whether and how those genes are activated is largely dependent on environmental factors. What you do, what you eat, where you go, when you sleep, and what you think all have an impact.

We humans may look like structures of skin, bone, muscle, and fat, but we are so much more. We are not just physical bodies, but also *energetic* ones. We are trillions of atoms and molecules that are teeming with potential. As we talk about bone broth and the breakthrough it can help facilitate for you long term, I want you to think of your body not as the sum of its parts, but as an enormous well of energy—so vast it could light up an entire city. Whatever you do in life that fuels that energy makes you healthy and vital and gorgeous.

When you think about fully living the bone broth lifestyle, I want you to approach it from the mindset that you are this matrix of energy, this dynamic confluence of cells, and those cells are constantly in motion—moving and changing to match your choices, your attitude, and your environment. How fitting that the word *matrix* goes back to the Latin for *womb*. You are a nurturing, supportive center for growth and renewal.

Renewal is key in this mindset. Almost every aspect of your biology works on a cycle. You breathe in and out. Your heart beats in constant rhythm. You sleep and wake. You eat, extract nutrients, eliminate waste, and start again. And throughout your body, cells are always in the process of cyclic turnover—which means that every day you're building the next new you. Talk about important work! You are clearing out weak, worn-out, sick cells and replacing them with healthy, strong ones. How? By creating an optimal internal environment during cellular turnover. Your cells have different lifespans, referred to as "generations." Red blood cells and white blood cells, for example, turn over every four months. Skin cells take one to two months to renew. Your bone cells take two to six years. Your intestinal cells take one to three weeks. That's why I made the original Bone Broth Diet a 21-day program—to give those critical cells a full cycle of cleansing, nourishment, and TLC as they renew.

Cellular renewal is a crucial factor for a flourishing long-term lifestyle because as each of your organs becomes refreshed through this process, your overall health keeps moving toward a new norm. It's like renovating your house, one room at a time—but this is your *body* you're renewing, your very health. And that's worth every second of effort you put into it.

Knowledge IS Power

When I was a kid, I loved a mystery. Or rather, I loved solving one. My parents used to call me Nancy Drew, and just like that beloved fictional sleuth, I'd scour the neighborhood with my pen and notebook, actively looking for things to figure out. If you're too young to remember Nancy Drew, think of me as Josh from *Blue's Clues*. Nothing made my day like helping a friend track down a lost dog or figuring out who was responsible for leaving a secret-admirer note. To be honest, the part of me that always wants to learn and understand has never gone away. It motivated me through school and college and biological medicine studies. I was constantly learning and making connections, deepening my understanding of how body and mind work—and work together. Sometimes it feels like learning is my oxygen.

In my practice, I tend to treat every patient's case as a new mystery. That's where my inner profiler gets to work. Figuring out the problem, creating a solution, watching things change for the better—it's such satisfying work. But if I am really doing my job right, I am also empowering each patient to become her own detective, to learn to recognize her body's clues and cues, to become an observant expert on her own habits.

Knowledge will be a critical part of your own transformation—of feeling confident you can live "off-diet" and continue to move toward your optimum weight (or toward maintaining it!), toward great skin and hair, toward your strongest and most energetic self.

How much of a difference can a little insight make? I meet people all the time who are doing everything they know to get healthy but are *still* struggling, still gaining, still feeling run down. I'm typically their last-stop doc, and so I know it's on me to help them figure out where things are going wrong. There are a few culprits I encounter again and again. Here are some repeat offenders:

- Believing some go-to part of a diet is healthy when it's doing a lot of damage. Hidden sugars, artificial sweeteners, and chemically loaded "health foods" are among the products that sneakily and frequently cause inflammation, which in turn takes a toll on all the body's systems. They're also major players in decimating your body's ability to get your blood sugar working for you instead of against you.
- Neglecting the body's need for sleep because of other more urgent priorities—a practice which almost always ends in a physical or emotional crash (or both).
- Being overweight but undernourished because of issues with the quality of your food or poor digestion of it.
- Operating every day highly caffeinated and stressed out—effectively shunting your body's real and extraordinary energy system. Over time, that approach wrecks your delicate hormonal balance, and then the dominos start to fall in the wrong direction as health problems compound one another.

Once you know the root of the problem, you can start confidently making changes that move you back toward harmony again. It takes time, but momentum breeds momentum, and it can keep tuning you up until you're exquisite again.

As a long-time student of ancient medicine, I can tell you that one theme through its histories all over the world is the power and undeniable appeal of knowledge. Throughout this book, I want to tap into the part of you that's already a sage, the part who's smart and savvy and constantly growing as a human being. That knowledge and that growth, those things are among your most powerful tools in getting a flat belly or shiny hair or a warm, sexy energy. They're also part of what makes you attractive and confident. Wisdom *is* sexy, and we're going to deepen both what you know and how you can use it in the coming chapters.

You Can Be Great at This

Did you ever work hard to learn a skill, like playing an instrument, speaking a language, being on a sports team, or taking dance classes? Or maybe you just had to relearn fourth-grade math or high-school geometry these past years to help your kids during virtual learning. You put in the work, got a handle on the fundamentals, and developed an understanding. Your fingers learned those scales, or you conjugated verbs until they were burned in your brain. You did ball-handling drills a thousand times, or you practiced your box step and turns until you could feel those motions in your dreams. After a while, you gained enough knowledge, enough mastery, to do those things automatically. Your body and mind knew what to do almost as surely as you know to breathe in and breathe out.

But what happened next? What I hope you experienced is a moment when you sat down at that piano or with your guitar and played something beautiful, just because you wanted to hear it. Or you carried on a conversation in a foreign language with fluency and glowed with pride. Or you jumped into a pickup game at a park and got lost in the joy of being a formidable, dynamic player. Or you danced at a wedding and felt so graceful, so in sync with your body, that it's a magical moment you'll never forget.

The same principles that brought you those kinds of moments are the ones that are going to make a lifestyle breakthrough both possible and sustainable. So much of this comes down to knowledge and practice in the beginning, which leads to habit, and then a lifestyle you can truly make your own.

Here's how we're going to approach the process: In chapter 2, we'll focus on the three basic truths that should be guiding our lifestyle choices. We'll look at how they're logical, scientific, and proven—and why it's ridiculously easy to ignore them in our modern world. In Part Two, we're going to delve into the essential building blocks of long-term diet, sleep, exercise, and self-care routines that will keep you healthy and strong as you figure out exactly what flourishing looks and feels like for you.

In each chapter, we're going to examine a few essential principles from every angle, and you're going to practice incorporating them into your daily life. Just like when you were taking those first piano or dance lessons, your body and mind are going to go through stops and starts of learning. You're going to make course corrections. There will be days when your steps feel clumsy and forced, but they'll be followed by days and then weeks where you understand that a positive transformation really is underway.

In Part Three, we're going to look at five common, persistent health snags that are so pervasive we all need to have a toolbox prepped to deal with them. All too often, these are the problems that derail otherwise healthy lifestyles. I'm going to show you how you can see each one coming, how you can nip it in the bud, and how you can feel strong and beautiful and confident once again by using bone broth as a foundational ingredient. I'm also going to share some amazing new recipes that are specifically designed to combat these problems—and how you can create more of your own using customized bone broths and condition-specific healing ingredients.

By the time we reach that point, I want you to have an attitude of, "I'm on this now. I'm making things happen." And I want you to know you're going to be successful in fully embracing and happily living your new lifestyle.

By the way, the longer you're successful at this lifestyle, the easier it gets. Some of that's just psychological: when you stick to something for a long period of time, it becomes a habit and the "easy" path for your brain to take. Another component, though, is cell-deep. After months and then years of maintaining weight loss and fostering healthy cell renewal, your body will find its way to a new normal—and it'll let go of the instinctive urge to get you back to your old, heavier, wearier self.

Chapter 2

Three Truths of Transformation

When I was a little girl, I spent a lot of time in my father's barbershop. My mom had four small kiddos at home, back to back, and let's face it—sending one of us off to hang out with Dad for a few hours made her life a whole lot easier. I lived for watching my dad work. He was confident and cheerful, and he had a knack for treating every customer as if they were the one person in the world he'd been hoping to see come through his door.

The thing that made the biggest impression on me was the transformation that happened when a customer sat in his barber chair. Time and again, I watched a client come shuffling into the shop, head down or eyes heavy, speaking softly or hanging back. But when he got up from the chair, he'd have pep in his step. He'd laugh and smile, shake my dad's hand, and walk out, head held high. Clearly, this was more than a haircut.

Watching my dad work provided my first insight into the fact that transformation is a big, layered process. Physical changes are the ones we can perceive at a glance, that tell us *this is something different*, but there's more to it. There's spark, there's swagger, there's underlying health, there's quiet confidence—all things that happen when you look great and feel strong.

Back in the day, my father's implements of change were scissors and razors, combs and hot towels, kindness and positivity. He knew that when somebody came to him, he had something special to give. It's been decades since I sat in the corner of that barber shop, but I still remember how it felt to witness those transformations. I like to think the work I do now is a continuation of that aspect of the "family business."

Some of the tools I work with are different, like medical science, nutrition guidance, and lifestyle advice—and some are the same, like compassion and kindness. One of the big approaches I share with my dad is doling out frequent (and occasionally unwanted) doses of unvarnished truth. If you are seeking or maintaining transformation, there's a part of me that'll always look at you like a good girlfriend does—believing in you, loving you for the work you're putting in, cheering you on. But I am equally a doctor, and in that role sometimes the most valuable thing I can offer is giving you direct and honest insight into what it's going to take to get where you want to be.

This is one of those times, because we need to get on the same page about big discrepancies between what our bodies need and the environment in which we live. The fact is, we are surrounded by beauty blockers, health blockers, and other factors that work against our overall well-being—and they are hiding in plain sight. Learning to recognize those blocks will help you take charge of the way you look and feel.

When you do? Transformations happen—weight loss and great skin happen, lustrous hair and smooth digestion happen, flat bellies happen. And attitudes change. Even people who once felt like they were sinking in quicksand start to rise, get air under their feet, and have pep in their step. Over my career, I've been lucky enough to play a part in thousands of these transformations, and the ones that make me happiest are the ones that are never going back. They've had the breakthrough, figured out the lifestyle, and made it part of who they are.

Let's talk about three truths that are far too easy to overlook—and far too important to ignore.

Truth #1: We Are Out of Our Element

Have you ever seen a creature living in an environment wildly unlike the one it was designed to inhabit? When I talk about this, I always think of a polar bear I once saw sprawled beside a warm, stagnant pool in a sweltering Florida zoo. Alone, belly-down on the concrete in her small enclosure, looking as wilted as a giant bear can possibly be. She was out of her element but surviving all the same.

What was happening to that polar bear was *adaptation*. Her body and mind had learned to adapt to the weather, the small space and the fence around it, the solitude, the warm pool instead of the open and cold sea, and the diet she was provided. She was probably on Prozac to help her come to grips with her lot in life (most polar bears in captivity are), but she was getting by.

At first mention, adaptation sounds like a good thing. We adapt to survive, right? That's pretty miraculous. In times of crisis, we can be faster, stronger, or braver than we ever thought possible in order to get through just about anything. But there's a dark side to those adjustments because if they are prolonged, they begin to take a negative toll on our bodies. The longer we're in that state, the more severe the consequences.

Take for example the elevated blood pressure and rush of adrenaline that helps you outrun a would-be mugger. That's a source of power for a few critical minutes. But what if you spend every day in a stressed-out, can't-stop state? Your body's hormonal balance goes off the rails. You accumulate fat. You suffer anxiety. Your skin dries and creases as if you're aging on fast forward. The very adaptation that saves your life in the short term can take years off it if you live like that for extended periods of time.

Hopefully you're not in the kind of dire straits that Miami polar bear was facing, but you do live in an environment that is less than ideal for you. Understanding this concept starts with a biological fact: Human DNA has been largely unchanged for more than forty thousand years.

But our world? Our world has changed explosively—the way we eat, the way we move (or don't move), the way many of us sleep, the way we view our relationship with our environment. We've undergone an agricultural revolution. An industrial revolution. A technological revolution. And our technological capability, which directly influences our daily realities, has doubled, and doubled, and doubled again.

In the center of this is you, engineered by tens of thousands of years of evolution to thrive in a natural environment but living in a world that constantly pushes things toward you that are detrimental to your health. You know what I'm talking about. Cake. Canola oil. Cola. Corn syrup. Twenty-four-hour streaming. Soy-based Frankenfoods. Binge drinking. Ten-hours-at-the-desk days. Incessant input from social media feeds. Blue light. Wi-Fi everywhere. The list goes on and on.

Let's look at how this plays out in just a few areas of our daily lives:

Diet

Our natural element: Simple meals from a selection of meats, eggs, fish, seasonal vegetables and fruits, a few nuts or seeds, and "good" fats like olive oil and coconut oil.

Our modern world: The average American supermarket contains over fifty thousand different foods. How many of them do you suppose are consistent with the diet our bodies are wired to digest? If I were a betting kind of girl, I'd wager you couldn't go to the grocery store and throw twenty packaged foods into your cart that aren't rife with sugar and chemicals (even though some of them would sport labels saying they are not).

Exercise

Our natural element: Remember, we are not just physical bodies but also energetic ones. Life is synonymous with movement. Look at your feet, your knees, your hips, your ribcage expanding and contracting as you breathe, your bendable spine, your nimble fingers. Every part of your miraculous body is designed to be in motion. When that happens, energy flows through you and throughout your cells.

Our modern world: We sit, sit, sit. The prevalence of sedentary jobs has increased over 80% since 1950. The number of jobs that are considered physically active has dwindled down below 20%. At home we've got Netflix with 24/7 programming designed to roll on, hour after hour, on the assumption that *we won't move*. In all of human history, we've never been as inactive as we are today.

Sleep

Our natural element: Every single thing about the body of a human adult is designed to go into slow mode when the sun goes down and to rev back up at dawn. During that time of rest, our system cleans house, heals, and preps for the coming day.

Our modern world: I can't tell you how often I meet women who are so tired they can barely function. When we talk about this crisis, conversations typically turn to all the other demands that are superseding sleep: work, kids, school, spouses, shopping, socializing, working out, housework. In a world where shift work, alarm clocks, phones in our hands, and light on demand abound, we've developed an almost total disregard for the circadian rhythms that have dictated when humans sleep for tens of thousands of years. Sometimes we even forget that sleep is just as essential to life as food or water.

. . .

So, what are you supposed to do about this giant gap between human nature and modern life? How do you keep your wits about you in a shiny, flashing world that's constantly offering opportunities to hit the pleasure button?

Right now, I am asking you to be mindful that you have needs your world does not automatically meet and that your lifestyle consistently presents you with things that aren't good for you. Knowing these things doesn't have to influence your every choice or action, but it should encourage you to routinely stop and ask the all-important questions: *Is this what I need? Is this good for me? Is this doing me harm? Is this pleasure worth its cost?* It's a simple gut check, a litmus test, but it'll shift your perspective. It'll allow you to make strategic choices. If you don't like the answers to those questions, take a step back and make new, *strategic* choices.

The change you make may be as small as drinking a big glass of water first thing each morning, taking a twenty-minute walk in the sunshine even though you've got a deadline looming at your desk, having bone broth as an ingredient in lunch, shutting down your kitchen after 7 p.m., or getting into your bed at 10:30 instead of midnight. The truth here is that we do have choices that support our well-being, but if we just float along in our modern world, we can easily forget to exercise them.

Truth #2: We Need to Focus on the Health of the House

We're lucky enough to live in a time when medicine can be miraculous. We have pharmaceuticals, therapies, and surgeries to help address almost any health crisis. This is such a blessing—one I'm grateful for every day.

But acute care and wellness care are not the same. Acute medicine is like the fire brigade. It comes barreling onto the scene with sirens wailing and pumps primed to put out the flames; it deals with your emergencies. Often, it provides you with adaptations that help make unacceptable conditions—like that high blood pressure—more tolerable.

What that kind of treatment does *not* do is improve the health of the proverbial house. Faulty wiring, poor insulation, a crumbling foundation—none of that changes when somebody puts out a fire. In fact, poor conditions can get even worse after a crisis and an intervention.

The truth is all our long-term lifestyle, beauty, and longevity goals are tied to something much bigger than just a lack of sickness. They're tied to consistent, deep-down cellular health. When you are truly well, your cells are flowing; they're hydrated, they're clean, and they're energized. So, what does it take to get those nurtured and healthy cells?

Optimal Nutrition

We're going to talk about this a lot in chapter 3, but one of the truths we need to agree about up front is that the better nourished you are, the better you'll look and feel. The human body is designed to absorb and utilize the molecules that make up nutrient-rich foods. This is the number-one thing to remember when you choose what you eat. It's the reason bone broth and other nutritionally packed superfoods are central to this lifestyle.

Equally importantly, there are foods that do nothing but irritate and aggravate your system. The popular modern diet of carbs, chemicals, sugars, and seed oils forces your system into that dreaded state of long-term adaptation—of constantly trying to cope with a bad situation. When your cells are healthy and well, think of them as a flowing river. When you fill your body with non-nutritious foods, you're damming up that river; you're polluting the water. And you're accumulating great quantities of useless waste that your body must accommodate (spoiler alert: one of the big ways it'll get this done is by putting down new layers of fat).

The truth is that diet is the single biggest determinant in the alchemy of cellular health.

Physical Activity

We all know we need to exercise, to move our bodies. But too often we don't, either because it can be draining or because we don't have the time. We need to agree that the effort to make this happen is worth it (and in chapter 5, we'll talk about ways to make it a more welcome part of your lifestyle). The benefits of movement are cell-deep throughout your body. For starters, getting a move on improves your body's uptake of oxygen. It supports the steady replacement of tired, old cells with new, healthy ones. It promotes blood flow and organ health. Movement begets movement, and the best way to get your cells humming with good health is to put your body in motion.

It's worth noting that all those outward signs of aging that we strive so hard to avoid are almost always present on the inside first. As our cells age, they struggle to divide, they get stagnant, and they start to feature misfolded and degenerating components. That's right—we have wrinkled, misshapen cells on the inside before we get them on the outside. Moving your body is the most powerful non-nutritional tool at your disposal.

Mindset

When I was seven, my dad joined a professional club called Dare to Be Great. For the same reasons my mom often sent me to the barbershop (mostly because I had a question for every minute of the day!), she sent me with him to those meetings. With a baby in her arms, she'd lay out my clothes on the bed, tell me to get dressed, and remind me to be polite and quiet at the meetings. This was, at its essence, a support group for people running businesses in our community. It was a center of *positivity* in my father's life—people who encouraged him, believed in him, and wanted him to succeed—and because I got to tag along, it was the same for me.

We don't talk about positivity enough. Countless studies and our own experience tell us that our thoughts and our words have power. What you believe and what you experience are inextricably tied together. A truth shared by nearly every successful and happy person I know is that they have learned to embrace what makes them unique and valued in this world. In my own life, I had to learn this one the hard way in order to reach the point where I stopped looking around at everybody else and instead looked inward. I had to make a very conscious decision to *like* being Kellyann, to love and accept the many different sides of myself.

If the idea of power in positivity sounds a little woo-woo to you, I promise I'll bring out the specific science to back it up in chapter 6. In the meantime, know that researchers at leading medical centers around the world are in agreement that there is a direct line between the way you feel and the composition and function of your cells. On a deep biological level, our feelings are actively modulating our health.

Truth #3: There Are Forces Working Against You

I wish this wasn't true. I really do. But I can tell you with certainty that on your way to any kind of self-improvement or transformation, you are going to encounter forces that are working against you. Don't let these forces sneak up or derail you. You can be prepared, and you can accomplish your goals despite subtle (and not so subtle) negativity.

Close to Home

I hope your circle of family, friends, and co-workers is full of the kinds of people who say, *Good for you!* and *I'm proud of you!* or even *I'll do it with you!* Chances are, though, there are also people in your life who somehow think that if you start sipping bone broth, or prioritizing me-time and sleep-time, or making your sandwiches on lettuce instead of bread that somehow means you're getting too big for your britches.

Here's what I want you to remember: If your growth is making someone around you uncomfortable, you have choices. If that person is on the periphery of your life, redraw the lines and put them squarely on the outside. Good riddance. But if they're too close or too important to cut ties with—and this happens all the time—you're going to have to choose not to be triggered. When somebody is directing their insecurity, jealousy, aggression, controlling nature, or gaslighting ways at you, you do *not* have to acknowledge, respond to, or even feel what they're offering. No matter what buttons they're trying to push, no matter how out of sync their words and actions are with the inner work you're doing, don't allot them any emotion. Have you heard of the "grey rock" method? It means becoming emotionally non-responsive—bland, cold, and unmoved. And it can be a very effective method of maintaining control of your situation.

When you are working to transform, when you start to achieve your goals, when you reach a point of feeling confident and strong and beautiful, I want you to find it within yourself to reject anybody's negativity. If your frenemy doesn't like that new dress that makes you feel like Cinderella (or J.Lo)? Grey rock. If an old pal thinks you're no fun because you only want one vodka cocktail instead of a slew of them? Grey rock. If your partner thinks that somehow your rediscovered good looks and confidence mean you're selfish or on the prowl? Well, it may be time to grey rock that person.

Taking care of yourself, practicing self-love, getting into the best shape of your life—those are goals and accomplishments that the people who really love you will celebrate with you. If they can't do that, you can either choose to help them understand, ignore their negativity, or push them a little closer to the edges of your life (or out of it entirely).

This concept has personal resonance for me. When I started achieving professional success, when I started taking better care of my body with the bone broth lifestyle, even when I decided I wanted to be blond instead of brunette—each change exposed people who were uncomfortable with me evolving. One of the hardest parts of transformation is realizing that when you start growing, not everyone will feel the positivity you're feeling or respond to the magnetism you're cultivating. In fact, sometimes it's quite the opposite. Some people only want the version of you they're familiar with—the old you. They look at you and see *change* rather than *growth*. Sometimes witnessing your transformation can even send someone you care about into a tailspin.

My best advice to you is *grow anyway*. Life is short. Aren't growth and purpose the point? Wear your crown while you're here.

Bad Companies

When it comes to making a long-term health breakthrough, the second kind of resistance you're likely to face comes from a wide swath of businesses and corporations that succeed when you fail. Sadly, much of the food industry falls into this category. In fact, they spend billions of dollars every year on marketing programs that are quite literally begging us to mistreat our bodies.

Think about it. We are constantly inundated with deliberate temptations to have a potato chip crunch-a-thon, an ice-cream social, a cake celebration, or a margarita moment. We are lured in with the promise of a treat—but the corporate objective is to market you into developing a habit in order to maintain their profits.

Consumers are studied up and down, inside and out. You are targeted in every possible way (and thanks to social-media marketing, some of those ways have gotten pretty intimate). Why? Because it's easier to get you to buy another bag of a salty, fatty, sugary, or borderline-addictive product than it is to get someone new to commit.

It's no wonder we get into trouble. It's no wonder so many people are going through this cycle day in and day out, indulging every night, feeling like hell every day. My goal is to raise your awareness of this constant and deliberate effort to manipulate your behavior for profit. The truth is, you are more than capable of fostering the kind of healthy perspective that keeps you in control of what you do, and do not, choose to eat.

Now that we're aligned in these three truths that help define a healthy mindset for your breakthrough, we need to turn our attention to the tools, tricks, and endless rewards of the bone broth lifestyle.

PART TWO

The Bone Broth Lifestyle in Action

et's talk about lifestyle—the things we do every day. Over the next four chapters, I'll lay out a baseline for what the break-through lifestyle looks like—simple daily steps to achieve and sustain health, beauty, and that je ne sais quoi that makes you shine. Later, in Part Three, we'll talk about some of the obstacles that can get in the way and how to move past them.

Transformations are my life's work, and after guiding them for more than twenty years, I've seen approaches that are a waste of time, some that work but aren't sustainable, and the ones that can fold seamlessly into our daily lives. Those are the gems—the lessons, meth-ods, and even hacks that help make our weight loss, great skin, and health achievements part of who we *are*, instead of just something we're working on.

In most cases, the things I'm asking you to do are what you do al-ready: sleep, eat, exercise, and take care of yourself—*but* I'm going to show you ways to shake up tired routines that aren't working and re-place them with new ones that offer a lot more reward for your effort.

Because routine is what it's all about, right? Your routines help de-fine your days, your days define your years, and your years define your life. The key to creating healthy, beautifying, lasting routines is leaning into what your body needs instead of ignoring or fighting its demands. The fact is, everything in our natural world is built on rhythms—the rotations of the earth, tides, sunrises and sunsets. Our bodies are just as rhythm-centric—sleeping and waking, eating and fasting, moving and being still, pushing our energy out into the world and then pulling back in to rest and recharge.

We've complicated these rhythms a whole lot with twenty-four-hour services, electricity and other energy on demand, and a mentality that we can just *force* our bodies to bend to our will. But look around at the people who are really thriving. Most of them have figured out how to work *with*—instead of *against*—their natural rhythms. Without all the friction of pushing your body to do what it doesn't want to do, you can truly get in tune with that best version of yourself.

Let's take a look at four of the most important elements of the breakthrough lifestyle: nutrition, sleep, movement, and what I like to call "stamina-care," and explore how you can both get in sync and thrive.

Chapter 3

Breakthrough Nutrition: Activate Your Body's Fat-Burning Power

I've written a number of books that have helped a lot of people lose weight, but I assure you that I don't just "do diets." Fact is, I look at every person and every situation in terms of overall health, not just the number on the scale! But I also know from experience that when you put the right foods into your body (and eliminate the wrong ones), you *do* look better and you feel better. It is not possible to underestimate the role of nutrition in wellness (or in fabulousness, for that matter).

Here's how I came to that realization for the first time in my life. From the age of twelve, I suffered from unbearable menstrual cramps—so bad I couldn't go to school; sometimes so awful I could barely get out of bed. I'd curl my body up around that pain and simply wait for it to end. It was a defining part of my teens, because for a week or more each month I was hurting so much I didn't know how to function.

My mom and I went to doctors asking for help, but those appointments were stressful and ominous. The doctors advised that I take birth control pills and plan to be on them for the rest of my life. I was prescribed pain medications that masked the discomfort but made me foggy. I was warned I'd probably never be able to have children—the one thing, as a little girl in a big Italian family, I'd been certain was in my future. More than once, I was told the only "cure" for my condition was a hysterectomy. I took none of this advice and continued to cope the best I could.

I now know that I had endometriosis, though I wouldn't learn that term for years. When I finally found relief from pain, it was thanks to a nutritionist who suspected there was a link between my monthly pain and my diet. He recommended I cut out dairy and gluten for a few weeks to see if that reduced my symptoms. My response? "What's *gluten*?" That's how little I knew back then about nutrition, about digestion, and about the way the body functions.

With an explanation in hand, I followed the plan. In just a few weeks, my shape was shifting—my waist leaner, my muscles taut. But something else was happening. The cramps I'd been living with since I hit puberty started to ease. A month passed without me spending a single day curled up on my bed. That sparked enough hope to keep me faithful to the new meal plan. By the third month, the discomfort that had been keeping me from living fully was gone.

To be clear, the pain that my doctors had told me could only be remedied by taking opioid drugs, by using permanent hormone therapy, or by undergoing a hysterectomy and forfeiting my hope of one day being a mom . . . was *gone*. It would be a while before the first studies would show that a gluten-free diet was clinically effective in eliminating endometriosis pain, but I was already living that truth.

As painful as those cramps were, I thank them every day for teaching me the method that would shape my entire career. *Diet matters.* Food can hurt, and food can heal. In my twenty years of seeing clinical patients in my own medical practice, time and again I've seen changes in diet help patients who were down and out get back on their feet and feel good again.

Never underestimate the power of being choosy about what you put into your body, because it can make a world of difference. If you want to lose thirty pounds? Look to your food. If you want to improve your mood? Look to your food. If you want to grow your hair or plump and soften your skin? Look to your food. And anytime you want to help your body move from sickness toward health? Look to your food to help you get there.

Easier said than done, I *know*. We don't so much choose this relationship as soak it up from our environment. In my big Italian family, I grew up eating carbohydrates—and often fried carbohydrates! Zeppole, pastas, seven fishes on Christmas Eve. I loved it all and didn't want to give it up or fear it. And, of course, now I know that a girl can't rock her je ne sais quoi if she feels anxious and fearful around food. If she can't feel powerful and comfortable enjoying meals, that's going to weigh her down and stress her out.

How do we fix our fraught relationship with food so it can help us heal, strengthen, and glow? How do we learn to eat healthy *and* enjoy?

This is where we start getting to the heart of the issue that keeps so many people, so many women, from reaching their ideal weight, their optimum health, and even from finding personal peace and happiness. Food is such a big part of our lives—an essential part—but not a day goes by that I don't hear from people who have tragically unhealthy relationships with it. They love it and hate it. They lust after it. They're ashamed to consume it. They get into miserable cycles of craving, indulgence, and regret. They think of everything they put in their mouths in terms of what's wrong with it and how sorry they will be once it's down the hatch.

Any of this sound familiar? If so, if I accomplish only one thing in these pages, I want to help you change your relationship with food. I want you to find joy in it. I want you to respect it. And I want you to know that diet can, and should, *serve* you and your health. I also want to be clear that even after—*especially* after—your relationship with food evolves, you'll still be able to indulge in and savor the foods that bring you joy (thanks, Marie Kondo).

This is the area of the breakthrough lifestyle where all of us most benefit from taking a step back to gain perspective. You've gotta eat. Being human means regular nourishment is a requirement for staying alive. Millions of people struggle with this simplest biological truth. This is not something to fight. It's something to embrace.

Let's take that one step further and acknowledge that food is meant to give us joy and comfort. Mother Nature doesn't fool around when it comes to ensuring the survival of a species. We are *wired* to want and to enjoy our meals (just like we're wired to want and enjoy sex). When we satisfy that need, we're rewarded with a surge of feel-good hormones—the same endorphins triggered by opioid medications. They whisper through the body, saying, *Yes! Great! Wonderful! Good job!* And they help us feel satisfied.

This is survival biology, so let's not feel ashamed of being hungry or relishing food. That's not the problem. The problem most of us face is that our modern, commercial world is in-your-face aggressive when it comes to food. This is an area where our completely healthy instinct to seek nourishment leaves us open to manipulation. We're bombarded day in and day out with temptation to eat ever-present products that barely deserve to be called *food*. Most chips, crackers, sweets, breads, muffins, and sodas (among others!) are pseudo-foods at best. They're fillers, literally filling you up, triggering your body's complex chemistry to falsely crave more.

Think of those healthy, feel-good hormones going rogue, whispering, *Again! Again! Again!*—driving you to overeat, to pack on extra weight, and to let your vibrant energy drain away. At the same time, they're putting your body chemistry on the fritz, these pseudo-foods take up space on your plate and in your body, leading you to skimp on the nutrition you need.

This, *not* weakness or lack of willpower, is the biggest reason we live in a time when it's astonishingly common for a person to be both overweight and poorly nourished.

A parallel problem is that many of us were conditioned to think that healthy food is unappetizing. Let's call it the tastes-like-cardboard complex. Here's the thing: that idea is a holdover from decades-old food guidelines that called for tons of grains and starches (six to eleven servings per day!) and virtually no fats. That's the 1992 FDA food pyramid for you, which has been debunked, dismissed, and rewritten many times over since it first came out. Despite a huge shift in the medical community toward more sensible paleo-centered guidelines, when I talk about eating nutritious foods, there are always folks who hear my words and picture a time when they watched their mother or their nana choke down a rice cake or a slice of whole-grain toast without butter.

I promise you my breakthrough nutrition plan is nothing like your nana's rice-cake diet. It's comprised of logical, practical guidelines and foods that are full of flavor—with enough options for you to have different, delicious meals every day of the year. In fact, in Part Three, I'll get you started by sharing dozens of flavorful, healthful new recipes that are so good you'll wonder where they've been all your life.

And here's another thing I'm very passionate about:

If you're at a weight you never thought you'd see on the scale . . .

If you have a health condition you never thought was in your future . . .

If trauma or a sick child or financial hardships left you struggling . . .

If you're in a place right now that you're not proud of . . .

. . . I want you to give yourself some grace. Taking one small, positive step today can be the beginning of your breakthrough.

The Basics of Breakthrough Nutrition

Step 1. Add Bone Broth

As if you didn't know that would be the first step!

Sipping bone broth is the equivalent of hosting happy hour for your cells. You can reap its benefits by incorporating two cups of this golden elixir into your diet every day. You can sip them straight or mix them into meals. If you happen to consume one or both of those cups in place of a sugary snack or drink—even better.

Bone broth is easy to make (but time consuming), and it's also readily available in grocery stores. Homemade is the gold standard because it both tastes great and is made from fresh ingredients. You'll find recipes for three basic broths on pages 271–75, as well as a number of custom, symptom-fighting versions in Part Three.

When time allows, I make my own, preparing enough for a week at a time. I enjoy the quiet concentration of cooking. But life is busy, and I can't always make time for that process. Thankfully, as the bone broth revolution roars on, there are also less time-consuming options available at almost any local market, including frozen, shelf-stable, and powdered versions.

If you buy pre-made (or ready-to-mix) bone broth, just know that stock (like chicken or beef stock) and bone broth are not the same food. These products usually sit right next to one another on shelves, and they look similar, but there's a giant disparity in their protein counts—regular broth typically has just a single gram per serving while bone broth sports 8 to 15 grams. It's the long, slow cooking process that makes the difference, as it pulls the nutrition right out of bones and ligaments.

Now let's talk about *why* bone broth is the cornerstone of this lifestyle, and why it's the ultimate transformative superfood.

Bone broth heals and seals your gut. An unhealthy gut is to your body what a radon leak is to your house. You can't see, smell, feel, or taste it, but it can nevertheless be the source of serious health consequences. An unhealthy gut is a giant problem, and many people who are living with it don't even know it. They don't realize it is taking a toll—playing a role in health issues they think are just a natural part of aging. We're talking about things like prematurely aging skin, thinning hair, stomach pain, constipation, a weak immune system, and even anxiety and depression. All of them can be caused or made worse by poor gut health.

The animal bones and connective tissues we simmer to make bone broth are loaded with collagen—the stuff that turns into gelatin when it's cooked. That gelatin is the reason your broth has heft and fills you up. It's also a balm to the lining of your gut. Think of it like aloe for a sunburn. It soothes irritation and promotes healing.

I can't overstate how important this is to foundational health and beauty. If your gut is healthy, you can eat a wider variety of foods without irritation. You're able to digest foods efficiently. If your gut is suffering, well, studies have linked poor gut health to everything from cardiovascular disease to cancer and irritable bowel syndrome to depression and diabetes. The scientific community is only just beginning to truly understand the critical role gut health plays in our lives, but every new study seems to reiterate that this is a vital, maybe even profound, piece in the puzzle of your overall well-being.

Bone broth offers deep hydration. Each serving of bone broth adds more liquid to your diet, sure, but this kind of hydration adds nutritional value that water and other liquids don't. Bone broth is loaded with minerals your body needs, among them calcium, magnesium, phosphorus, potassium, and sodium. These and other vital nutrients replenish your body's electrolytes—without all the real or artificial sugars of sports drinks.

Bone broth nourishes your skin. Bone broth is rich in collagen, a nutrient that plumps skin, erases lines and wrinkles, and thickens hair. Studies have documented its effectiveness in increased expression of genes associated with skin and hair development. Translation? If you can get collagen into your body in a form it can utilize—it is truly a fountain of youth.

Bone broth can improve joint health. The gelatin that comes from cooking bones contains three of the most important therapeutic ingredients for good joint health: glucosamine, chondroitin, and hyaluronic acid. These are essential components of many physicians' arthritis treatment regimens, and many bone broth devotees report losing those aches and pains in hips, ankles, knees, and other joints.

Bone broth contains a natural key to good sleep. Research tells us that ingesting glycine, one of the amino acids in gelatin, before bed helps people sleep better. Sometimes this is the benefit of bone broth that surprises my patients the most! They expect to look better and to lose weight. They hope to have more energy. But few dare to dream they'll be able to sleep like babies again.

Bone broth helps detoxify your body. In addition to all its other benefits, the rock star we know as glycine is also an essential building block of glutathione. And what's that? It's a powerful antioxidant. In fact, my friend Dr. Mark Hyman calls glutathione "the mother of all antioxidants." Every cell in your body contains this miracle worker, and part of the work it does is recycling your other antioxidants so they can go back to work scrubbing toxins out of your system. So, while you're sleeping, your bone broth continues to cleanse your body.

Bone broth helps you stretch the time between meals. Dietary scientists have an ever-growing mountain of evidence that tell us strategic, small fasts are powerful tools for weight management (more about that in step 4). The problem, of course, is that fasting can make us feel tired, depleted, and miserable. Bone broth is a huge problem solver for anybody who wants to fast but suffers getting through it. You can sip it *while fasting*, it has more density and flavor than water or tea, and it's packed with nutrients that will help your body feel satisfied, even while you're incinerating fat.

Getting bone broth into your diet offers benefits to make it worth your while—no matter what else you eat.

How much bone broth is enough to make a difference?
Shoot for 2 cups each day!

More Gut-Cleansing Foods

Bone broth is truly a power cleanser for your cells, but it's not the only one. The fact is we need all the help we can get to keep our cells working optimally. The food we eat, the air we breathe, the water we drink—they're all dirty with environmental toxins, so I recommend working in as many nutrient-rich, gut-cleansing foods as you can into your diet. Think of these supercleansers like a bingo game: How many can you bring into your diet over the course of a week?

- Collagen: This is a key ingredient of bone broth, but it's also a nutrient you can find in other forms, including supplements easily added to coffee, smoothies, and meals.
- Citrus fruits: Lemons and grapefruit flush toxins like crazy and offer a powerful vitamin C boost. I'm a huge fan of starting each morning with a glass of hot lemon water—it's a perfect way to kick off the day's hydration (without breaking your overnight fast), kick-start your metabolism, and get that cellular cleansing underway.
- Beets: Beets increase the liver's production of bile and reduce inflammation—the first step in healing anything that's going haywire in the body.
- Dandelion: So much more than just a weed! Dandelions boost your liver's detoxing abilities. You can toss these greens into salads or soups, take dandelion in capsule form, or drink dandelion tea.
- Garlic and onions: These two sulfur-rich foods are vital antioxidants that latch onto toxins and escort them out of your body. They're especially useful for flushing out heavy metals and protecting you against kidney damage, as well as colon and liver cancers.

- Cruciferous vegetables (broccoli, Brussels sprouts, cauliflower, cabbage, kale, radishes, and watercress): X marks the spot on these wonder foods—literally. They get their name from a root word that means "cross-bearing" because they bloom in four symmetrical petals. These veggies are loaded with natural compounds that fight inflammation and protect your body from damaging toxins.
- Turmeric: This "gold-rush spice" pairs with both sweet and savory foods, reduces inflammation, reduces blood sugar, and encourages brain cell growth. This superstar of the spice cabinet comes from a gnarled root, and people have been using it for over four thousand years for flavoring and medicine. You can add it to bone broth, stews, casseroles, and curries—but also to applesauce, oatmeal, and tea. It's available fresh in many produce aisles, as well as dried in the spice aisle and in capsules in the supplement section of your grocery store.
- Avocado: What can't avocado do? This superfood is so effective at nourishing your body and brain, and it's also a beauty booster that moisturizes and smooths your skin from the inside out. It's easy to forget it's also an excellent source of detoxifying glutathione.

Step 2: Eat!

Now it's time to eat. It's so plain and simple that I didn't even waste time writing a pithy title for this step. Why? Because I'm sick and tired of deprivation diets. You have to nourish your body. And I want you to eat real, recognizable foods. I want you to think about building a robust plate at every meal.

A 200-calorie protein bar will never nourish you the way a 200-calorie plate of zucchini noodles with olive oil, fresh tomatoes, and basil will.

A 300-calorie frozen diet meal will never satisfy you the way a sweet potato with pasture-raised butter and a beef patty will.

Before you plan any meal, I want you to ask yourself three questions:

1. What about this dish will nourish me?
2. Will it give me everything I need?
3. What about it will make me happy?

Most of the time, your plate should consist of the same major elements: protein, fat, two kinds of veggies (more on that in a minute), and sometimes fruit. If you think that sounds boring or unappetizing, you're not truly considering the possibilities. Picture your plate like one of those four-digit electronic locks. On a lock where there are only nine single digits for each slot, there are ten thousand potential combinations. Your dietary choices are far wider. There are an infinite number of ways to compose a plate that meets your nutritional requirements—*and also tastes delicious.*

Putting it all together is a flexible process, but a good target for most meals is to include 1 to 2 servings of protein, 1 to 2 servings of fat, 1 generous serving of fibrous vegetables, and 1 serving of starchy vegetables. A serving of fruit can be incorporated in the meal, but I prefer to have mine for snacks and in desserts.

Healthy Proteins

Proteins create structural support in cells, strengthen and repair muscles, transport molecules and messages, and are the catalysts for thousands of biochemical reactions taking place in your cells. They are the dietary workhorses of your body's systems. They include: beef, poultry, fish, shellfish, wild game, eggs, organ meats, MSG-free jerky, nitrate- and nitrite-free deli meats and sausages.

Buy better: When it comes to meat, buy the best you can afford, focusing on pasture-raised and free-range, as well as organic. At a cellular level, animals raised in feedlots on corn and antibiotics are fundamentally different from those that roam pastures eating grass.

Portion it out: A single serving should be no bigger than the size and thickness of your palm.

Healthy Fats

Believe it or not, it wasn't until 2015 that the committee in charge of Dietary Guidelines for Americans *finally* saw the light and dropped its restrictions on dietary fat. Healthy fats are critical to your overall health, gut health, and brain health, and they also play a starring role in creating the beautiful skin we've been talking about.

I told you this is not your nana's nutrition plan! Healthy fats include: avocado oil, coconut oil, ghee, grapeseed oil, pasture-raised butter, macadamia oil, olive oil, avocado, coconut chips, olives, almond butter, chia seeds, ground flaxseed, hemp seeds, nuts.

Buy better: Keep in mind that pasture-raised butter is fundamentally more nutrient-rich than butter from grain-fed cows. It has more vitamins, a far better ratio of omega-3 to omega-6 fatty acids, and includes a powerful inflammation-fighting fatty acid. I know buying pasture-raised means going deeper into your pocket at the grocery store, but I believe its benefit to your body is worth the investment. For nuts and seeds, choose raw and unsalted whenever possible.

Portion it out: A serving of oil, ghee, avocado, nuts, or other approved fats is about the size of your thumb, or 1 to 2 tablespoons.

Fibrous Vegetables

Green and colorful veggies—they are the rainbow of nutrition that makes us healthy, strong, and attractive. I could list them all for you, but it's simpler to note the veggies that do *not* fall into this category: beets, carrots, corn, legumes, potatoes of all kinds, pumpkin, and squash. There's a place for most starchy veggies in your life, but because of the way your body digests them and utilizes their nutrients, they belong in a separate food category.

Buy better: Opt for seasonal, local, and/or organic veggies when you can. They are always a step up from their out-of-season, shipped-in, and pesticide-treated counterparts. Prioritize buying organic collard and mustard greens, kale, peppers, spinach, and tomatoes. The Environmental Working Group's extensive research consistently finds that these are the most heavily contaminated veggies in the produce section.

Portion it out: Go big! A single serving is about the size of a softball.

Starchy Vegetables

These are what I like to call the "slow carbs" because they elevate your blood sugar in a low, steady fashion. They're a power source without the spike-and-crash impact of sugary sweets. Starchy vegetables include: beets, carrots, green peas, parsnips, plantains, potatoes, pumpkin, squash, sweet potatoes, turnips, yams.

Buy better: Choose organic when you can, especially when it comes to potatoes. You can peel them to remove a good portion of any pesticides, but this means wasting a lot of the valuable fiber and potassium instead of consuming it!

Portion it out: About $1/_2$ cup per meal.

Fruits

Small quantities of fruits every day broaden the range of vitamins and nutrients your body gets and fill you with healthy doses of feel-good hormones. We all want a little sweetness in our lives, and the good green Earth is happy to provide: apples, apricots, bananas, berries, cantaloupe, cherries, cranberries, grapefruit, grapes, honeydew, kiwi, kumquats, lemons, limes, lychees, mangoes, nectarines, all kinds of oranges, papayas, peaches, pears, pineapples, plums, pomegranates, watermelon, and others.

Buy better: Buy the freshest seasonal fruit you can find. Whenever possible, choose organic, especially when it comes to berries, cherries, grapes, peaches, apples, and nectarines. These are typically the fruits most contaminated by pesticides.

Portion it out: About $^1/_2$ cup, up to twice a day.

Reading Labels, Front and Back

Remember the terrible haircut called the mullet? Business in the front, party in the back? I want you to think of that haircut when you read a food product label.

When it comes to food packaging, the party's in the front—all the splashy logos, the bold marketing claims, the beautiful photos. Every inch of that packaging is designed to catch your eye and stimulate your appetite. In the back? That's where you find the business side—the nutritional facts. So please, flip that food packaging over and get to know what's really in your food. Here's what to look for, all qualities you can assess in a few seconds:

- Look for products with the fewest ingredients—half a dozen or less is great, though there are exceptions (especially for lists of spices). In general, less is more.
- Look for ingredients you can pronounce and picture in your mind, foods that originate in nature rather than on a conveyor belt. Tomato? Check. Onion? Check. Salt? Okay, if it's not too much. Soy lecithin? Um, no. Maltodextrin? Not for me, thanks. Think about it this way: if you don't recognize it, there's a decent chance your body won't be able to recognize it either.
- Look for, and avoid, the sugar, corn, and oil trap. Certain ingredients are terrible for our bodies and we know it. Sugar, corn,

wheat, high-fructose corn syrup, palm oil, monosodium gluta-mate (MSG)—each of these should make you pause and ask yourself, *Do I really want this crud in my system?*

- Look for the sneaky crooks—a lot of unhealthy ingredients have aliases. So many, in fact, that it can be a challenge to keep track of them all. For example, there are over one hundred pos-sible names for sugar (you can identify a lot of them by the "-ose" on the end: fructose, glucose, lactose, sucrose, and so on). You can find an exhaustive list of these aka ingredients at DrKellyann.com.

- Look for portion size—before you can understand the nutri-tional information (aside from the ingredients), you've got to know the serving size. Food manufacturers are clever at mis-leading you. Examples include servings that are half of an individual-size snack pack, half a can of soup, half a cup of ice cream, and tablespoon-size portions of condiments most peo-ple eat at least twice as much of. Also look closely at nuts, gra-nolas, and trail mix. Snacky things are so easy to overindulge in, especially from a big bag, so measure from time to time to be sure you know how much you're eating. All the information on a label is based on the serving size as determined by the com-pany, so be sure you know what it is.

- Look for the box score—the first group of nutrients listed are ones you want to try to limit in your daily diet. Fat, saturated fat, trans fat, cholesterol, and sodium are all best consumed in small amounts (or in the case of trans fats, not at all if you can help it.

  The second group of nutrients are ones that are typically not consumed enough in American diets. In this list, you'll find essential nutrients, such as iron, calcium, dietary fiber, vitamin A, and vitamin C.

- Want to spend less time reading labels? The simplest hack, one I live by, is finding brands you know and trust. Once you know a brand shares your food values, you won't have to scrutinize every inch of every label to get to the truth. My personal list is always changing (and growing, because more companies are making commitments to responsible practices!). At this writing, these are a few of the brands I've come to love and trust:
  - Primal Kitchen for sauces, condiments, and frozen foods with no gluten, grain, sugar, or industrially processed oils.
  - Steve's Paleo Goods for grain-free, moderate-carb snacks.
  - Siete for snacks that are free of grain and industrial seed oils.
  - Coconut Secret for organic, gluten-free, and soy-free condiments and sauces.
  - MALK Organics for organic unsweetened almond milk that's free of gums, fillers, oils, and gluten.
  - Elmhurst for unsweetened nut milks that are free of gums, fillers, oils, and gluten.
  - Cappello's for pastas that are gluten-free, grain-free, soy-free, and dairy-free.
  - Native Forest for canned coconut milk with no gums or preservatives.
  - Lynn's Life for bread mixes and crackers with no grain, sugar, gluten, or dairy.

Step 3: Automate

No one has time to plan three meals and two snacks *and* save the world each day. I know the information I just gave you was a *lot*. That's why I recommend automating two meals a day anytime you feel like planning is too much. This works wonders in a busy schedule.

Automate your meals as often as you find helpful. This means figuring out a couple of meals—a lunch and a dinner, say—that you can prepare ahead of time and grab whenever you're short on time or patience. When you get bored with the ones you've been eating regularly, choose new ones to shake up the routine.

This works especially well for anybody who makes soup or another big meal on the weekends. Just portion out the week's worth of food, and you can grab and go. In Part Three, you'll see I've been on quite a soup kick myself—there are plenty of new healthy and yummy recipes to try there.

Besides saving time, this method removes some of the on-the-spot food choices from the equation. When you think of times your healthy eating agenda gets derailed, chances are most of them are when you didn't plan or were in a hurry. This approach to daily eating gives you guardrails.

This is yet another reason why I'm so passionate about bone broth—it's automated. You can have it anytime, on its own or with any meal. It provides a generous dose of nutrients, and it soothes and restores your body. If you're in a hurry, out of ideas, or just too tired to bother sorting out a meal plan, a bowl of bone broth (with or without any nutritious proteins, fibrous veggies, or healthy fats you have on hand) is a can't-go-wrong meal option. If you follow any of my social media accounts, you'll notice that I do this *all the time*. I simmer a little bone broth, add salmon, any diced vegetable, and half an avocado. And just like that, I've got a healthy, filling, delicious meal.

Step 4: Lose (or Reduce) Gut-Wrecking Beauty Blockers

Let's face facts: There are a lot of items among the fifty-thousand-plus options at your grocery store that Mother Nature never intended for humans to eat. In fact, I suspect that if she ever got a look at an Oreo or a bag of Cheetos, her head would spin. I know I sometimes think mine is going to.

The trouble with these foods is that a handful of deeply unhealthy ingredients are underpinning most of them. No matter what color, shape, taste profile, or food group, chances are any packaged food you pick up that isn't explicitly labeled as *not* containing sugar, industrial seed oils, and gluten in their many forms is largely constructed of the three of them.

It's no wonder we live in a time when a majority of Americans are overweight or obese. We need this knowledge—and to act on it—to maintain our good health. These foods do a lot of harm and very little (if any) good, so avoid them when you can.

Sugar

If you want to cut the one thing from your diet that will make the biggest difference, look no further than sugar. Picture the inside of your body as smooth and soft. Your cells glide along in this pliant, delicate home. Sugar is like ground glass in that vessel. It is abrasive and destructive to almost everything it touches. It rollicks through your body, wreaking havoc. Over time, it ages your skin. It interferes with your ability to burn fat. It teaches your body to ignore the natural signals that tell you when you're hungry and full. It inflames your arteries. It strains your kidneys. It decays your teeth. It impairs your memory and puts you at higher risk for heart disease, Alzheimer's disease, and cancer.

Shall I continue?

I know this is a tough subject for a lot of people because the average American adult gets roughly 17% of a day's calories from sugar. That's a lot to cut out—especially when you start looking at where that sugar is coming from. If you only consumed the sugar you spooned into your coffee and mixed into homemade desserts, you might hit four or five teaspoons a day. But studies show most of us are getting roughly *five times* that much. That's because it's *hidden* in breads, cereals, beverages, condiments and sauces, and just about every other processed food in your pantry.

Do you have to give it up completely? You should. We all should. But that's a high bar. Not only do we love the taste of it, we love the role it plays in our communities and rituals. I am not suggesting you can't—or even shouldn't—have a piña colada on your vacation, or a slice of cake at a wedding, or ice cream with your kids on a hot summer day. I'm suggesting you eat *less* sugar, as little as you possibly can. I can tell you from experience that my patients who chose to do this have reaped the rewards of that sacrifice in every other area of their lifestyles. They turn back the aging clock, they reclaim glowing skin, their eyes sparkle, they sleep better, they lose weight, they have more energy, and they report being more clear-headed—sometimes for the first time in years.

When we look at other common dietary irritants like grains, gluten, and dairy, there's often a continuum in terms of the damage they do. Some people can't tolerate them at all, others have mild problems but can eat them in moderation, and some seem to manage them just fine. But to be clear, sugar is a toxin for everyone.

Artificial Sweeteners

I'm hoping you gave these up long ago (or just never started consuming them in the first place), but since there were entire generations of us who had this pushed our way as a "healthier" alternative to sugar, it can't be left unsaid. These additives have no benefit. They wreak havoc on your blood sugar just like the sugar demon does. You don't need this daily dose of chemicals.

When you're cutting out sweeteners, it can feel like they're leaving a big hole in your diet. The best way to optimize your health is to white-knuckle your way past those cravings, but I realize that may not work for you. If you're looking for alternative foods that aren't as damaging to the body, coconut, date, and palm sugars; raw honey; maple syrup; 100% fruit jam; apple juice concentrate; applesauce; dates; smashed bananas; blackstrap molasses; and green leaf stevia are all healthier options.

Grains

I'm sure you noticed that there were no breads, crackers, rice, or other grains among the foods I recommend for breakthrough nutrition. There are good reasons for that. Like gluten and dairy, grains are ingredients *some* people can eat without troubles, but many cannot. The big problem is that these foods could be damaging your gut and creating inflammation in your body, and all the while you might be blissfully unaware it's happening. This is the reason I recommend that even if you don't eliminate this food entirely, you keep it to a minimum.

The trouble with grains is rooted in our lack of suitability to process them. Humans have been eating grains only since the advent of agriculture, about ten thousand years ago. It's a long time, but not long enough for evolution. We can grow these foods, but that doesn't mean we come equipped with the necessary chemical tools to process them. Your gut gets those grains and asks (every time), *What the heck is this?*

Certain foods go into your body like a key custom made for a lock—they're a perfect fit, and the lock knows exactly what to do with it. Grains are the ill-fitting key in the lock of your digestive system. It'll go through, sure, but the force and irritation it takes to make that happen may just damage the entire apparatus.

The disruption grains cause carries on throughout your digestive process. They interfere with the absorption of vitamins and minerals from other foods, sapping your body of nutrients. They also spike your blood sugar, creating many of the same "ground glass" effects as refined sugar.

Gluten

Gluten is the natural protein that gives grains their doughy, spongy texture. Isolated from grains, gluten is commonly used as a stabilizer to thicken and bind a vast array of foods, ranging from sauces and condiments to gums and candies, from chips and cold cuts to flavored rice and crackers. Even beer hasn't escaped gluten's long, sticky reach.

Like grains, gluten is a food product that a lot of people are reactive to and they don't even know it. The consequences of gluten sensitivity are centered in the gut, where it can cause something called "intestinal permeability." In the simplest terms, this means the walls of your gut are weakened and allow nutrients and irritants to pass through willy-nilly, upsetting not just your digestive system but every other part of your body as irritation and nutritional deprivation ensue.

Because of my own life-changing experience with cutting out gluten, and because I have seen similarly dramatic changes play out with hundreds of patients over the years, I recommend that everyone—even if your nutrition plan is all about flexibility and forgiveness—take a "gluten retreat." Give it up for three weeks, and then slowly add it back into your diet. If you don't notice a difference, no harm, no foul. Have a roll with dinner. But if you are one of the estimated third of adults who are highly sensitive to this food, you may find giving it up makes your whole world better.

Dairy

This is yet another secret offender—a food most people eat and, in my experience, a majority have troubles with. You may be wondering how this could be a problem—after all, humans have been eating dairy for ages. That's true, but a significant number of those people, from thousands of years ago right up until today, have significant trouble digesting it. Sometimes the problem is severe enough that the individual eventually puts together the fact that dairy equals trouble (especially bloating). But others go through their lives with all kinds of niggling inflammations and irritations and simply believe that's their normal.

That's why when I ask my patients to take a three-week break from dairy, they are often stunned by the changes in their bodies. Me? I'm never surprised. Nutrition specialists see all the time that when clients cut dairy, their acne, allergies, or bloating magically disappear at the same time.

Step 5: Intermittent Fasting Hack

In the last decade, one of the most important and impactful changes in how people think about nutrition is the realization that *when* you eat matters almost as much as *what* you eat. If you've done any of my diets, you know that I am a huge fan of intermittent fasting for this reason.

Giving your body a break between meals allows your digestive system and your entire cellular being to process, rest, and heal. And depending on how you implement it, this practice can help you lose weight or maintain the losses you've already made.

Why does it matter if you're eating or not? Because digestion is hard work. While your body is engaged in that process, a significant portion of your energy is directed toward it. And we are not genetically wired to be doing that work all the time. Think about your ancestors. How many of them do you suppose ate three square meals and grazed all day? How many kept eating for hours after the sun went down? Bringing home every meal through your own effort out in the wild would make that kind of nonstop dining nearly impossible. We evolved to eat and then to not eat for a while as we looked for our next meal. Simple.

To return to this lost way of eating, you can adopt intermittent fasting (which is one of the easiest health hacks) into your life, and it does not have to be a sacrifice. In fact, after they get the hang of it, most people who start down this path love being on it. Like me, they sleep better when they're not still digesting their last meal of the day—and they love that empty-belly feeling in the morning.

Just to be clear, we're not talking about forty days and forty nights here. We're not talking about anything even remotely dramatic. There are a lot of ways to get the job done that will barely change your day. As part of the breakthrough lifestyle, I recommend setting a daily rhythm that confines your meals to a period of eight hours or so.

So, you might adopt an 8/16 pattern where you eat your meals during the eight hours between 10:00 a.m. and 6:00 p.m., then abstain for sixteen hours until 10:00 a.m. the next morning. If that's too long for you, it's not a problem. Try a 10/14 pattern instead, widening that eating window from 9 a.m. to 7 p.m. If you have a day with an event or even just a movie night and don't want to stick to the program, that's fine. The bone broth lifestyle is all about what you do *most of the time.* The important thing is to respect a natural cycle of eating and then give your digestive system a rest.

Bone broth is absolutely key here because it *does not count* as food in your fast. If you need a pick-me-up in the morning or the evening, sip to your heart's content. If you're prone to feeling weak during even a short fast, the bone broth will help keep your blood sugar from going haywire.

The simple act of organizing your days so that your meals fall into this kind of eating and fasting pattern brings rewards in many forms. First, it's an amazing tool for weight maintenance. If you're trying to lose, be a little more restrictive or add one full-day fast to each week. While you're doing these little fasts, your body will be hard at work doing housekeeping tasks like detoxing your cells, repairing your gut, and building your muscles.

A quick note about those eating hours to remember (because every once in a while, I meet someone who thinks eating *during* eight hours means eating *for* eight hours): During the day, even during that eight- or ten-hour window, the time you spend *not* eating is as crucial as the time you spend eating. Your body can't burn fat when your blood glucose is high and you're still circulating insulin to deal with a meal you ate hours ago. If you're tempted to graze between meals, enjoy a mug of bone broth instead.

The rest of the time, when you're eating, be *eating*. Sit down, focus on your meal, chew thoroughly and slowly, and most of all, enjoy. Between meals and planned snacks, focus your mind and body on other things.

Rethinking Break-Fast

Here's an effective pro tip from my years of transformation work: don't get hung up on breakfast being first thing in the morning.

I know your mother probably said this was the most important meal of the day, but I'm telling you there is a mountain of research-based evidence telling us that extending the period between your last meal in the evening and your first of the next day gives your body a chance to heal and rest. Instead of viewing breakfast as the thing you do as soon as you start moving in the morning, view it in terms of its literal meaning: breaking your fast. For me, 11 a.m. is a great time to start eating. If I get hungry before that, I'm happy with a cup of bone broth to hold me over. That late breakfast time means I go about my morning with a feeling of purpose I've come to really appreciate.

When you do break the fast, you'll need to disregard another old adage about healthy nutrition: the one that says breakfast should be cereal, toast, or a muffin—just one big grain fest. Your body doesn't need grains at all, and it certainly doesn't need them for your first meal of the day.

Instead, breakfast is the perfect time to give your body what it most needs: protein and healthy fat. Try two eggs and half an avocado and see how you feel!

Step 6: Hydrate

Water is life! It is the most essential part of your body. Everything is connected to it. It helps regulate your body temperature, transport nutrients and oxygen into your cells, and carry toxins away from them. When you don't get enough? Your energy drops, your mood gets irritable, your cells are sluggish, you get headaches. And against simple logic, you get bloated because your body desperately clings to the water it does have.

Hydration is also imperative for brain function. In a study where participants exercised until their hydration level was down to just 1 to 3%, their concentration, problem-solving ability, and coordination were all measurably depleted. Shortcomings like that can easily translate into mistakes, accidents, feeling poorly, or snapping at your kids or co-workers.

There's a lot of debate about how much water we need—and with variables like age, weight, climate, and activity involved, there is no one-size-fits-all chart (nor is there a well-researched universal recommendation). In my experience as a clinician, a great baseline recommendation is to follow this simple formula: take your body weight in pounds, halve it, and drink that number in ounces. Most of my patients find that drinking that amount of water each day keeps them well hydrated.

I get a lot of questions about what does and does not count toward this hydration goal, so here's a rundown.

- Temperature doesn't matter. Drink your water piping hot or ice cold—as long as you drink it.
- Carbonated water and flavored water are just as good as still water (as long as they're not full of additives or sugars).
- All liquids except alcohol and sugary drinks count. Yes, you can count your black coffee toward your quota. Tea also counts. And, of course, bone broth counts.
- Not loving to drink water is, unfortunately, not a good enough reason

to not drink it. You can kick up its flavor in countless ways to make it more palatable. These are a few of my favorites:

- Squeeze in a wedge of lemon, lime, or orange
- Soak in herbs like fresh mint, basil, or cilantro
- Add melon, berries, or pineapple to create a cocktail-like experience (double the fun by adding them to sparkling water)
- Add cucumber slices to create a spa-style flavor

Love That Lemon Water

Bone broth will always be my Number One, but next in line is warm lemon water. I start every morning with a glass of this simple, powerful combo. Lemons are low in sugar but bursting with nutrients. They give you vitamin C, riboflavin, folate, calcium, iron, magnesium, and vitamins B_6, A, and E. Because of all that action, this morning cocktail doesn't just give you a much-needed kick-start to the day's hydration. It also works to purify your body, boost your immune system, support healthy digestion, and reduce your risk of kidney stones. Cheers!

80/20, Baby!

The programs I design are for health. I know I've packaged some of them as 5-, 10-, or 21-day programs, but I admit I'm a little sneaky there. My goal is always to steer readers toward the tenets in this book—the tenets of bone-deep, long-term health. The thing all my programs have in common (besides bone broth, of course) is that they're working toward three primary goals:

- Reducing inflammation
- Healing the gut
- Training your body to be a fat burner

If you follow the steps in this plan, all three will happen, and yeah—you'll get healthy. You'll also get fewer chins, less arm flab, a smaller waist, better skin, brighter eyes, less gas and bloat, less fatigue, better sleep, and a sex drive that may have been MIA for a long time. That's just how it works when you do the work.

My goal here is to help you set positive goals to take you down this road. It's about the things you do, the things you want, and the things you get. It's absolutely *not* about statements that start with "I never," "I can't ever," or "I have to." You don't *have* to do anything!

And of course, this is the sticky part of every healthy nutrition plan—the part where I'd love to tell you that it's okay to have all the wine, lasagna, and ice cream you like while you're living life to the fullest. Truly. We all know it doesn't work that way. Odds are you have someone in your life who has chosen to go down this path, and you've seen the health damage the all-you-can-eat-or-drink approach does in the long term. Decadent eating and drinking begin to weigh you down if you choose to live that way every day.

But there is an in-between—a happy place between decadence and deprivation. And I hope we can all agree that it's *fine* to have wine, ice cream, a donut, or a slice of pizza—sometimes. Every single word of my nutrition lifestyle advice is designed to be applied *most of the time*. Why? Because we're all perfectly imperfect. We're not robots. Sometimes we just want something and choose to have it. Sometimes we get caught up in a glorious or miserable moment and indulge.

I'll let you in on a secret: As a concierge doctor to actors, models, movies stars, musicians, and some ridiculously beautiful people, I've had a seat at some fascinating and very fancy tables. These are people the camera loves, who look good in swimsuits—even up close. They're the ones who dazzle everyone in their orbit with their looks and energy. Guess how many of them are 100% on their nutrition plans? None. Nada. Nobody. Even the healthiest, even the skinniest, even the most toned and sculpted among us break protocol sometimes. And that's okay.

A good guideline for a balanced lifestyle is an 80/20 target: For 80% of meals, stick to nourishing, satisfying (and delicious) foundational foods—everything on my lists of proteins, vegetables, healthy fats, and fruits. The other 20% of the time, sprinkle what I like to call "fairy dust foods" into the mix. What's your fairy dust? For some people it's a favorite dessert, a cheeseburger, or a bowl of rocky road. It's all okay. If you manage your portion sizes, you don't need to make any food off-limits.

Here's another secret: It may feel like the right and moderate step to indulge in those 20% foods a little every day, but that's not true. If you have to choose between, say, a quarter cup of ice cream every night or a pint on Sunday, the one-day splurge will do less damage to your gut health and your weight than the every-day treat. Why? Because it's easier for your body to be a fat burner, have a healthy gut, and manage inflammation if it's not endlessly having to deal with an ice-cream drip.

I will warn you that after eating mostly lean proteins, fibrous veggies, and healthy fats for a while, you may be surprised to find the things that were once your favorite splurges—those sugar/fat/sodium/gluten/dairy bombs—have lost some of their appeal. When your body's nutritional needs are met and your gut is healthy, a lot of cravings for sweet, salty, or fatty foods start to recede. No matter what, however, you should never beat yourself up about making a dietary choice—even if it's for something less than great for you.

My philosophy on this is simple: We are talking about lifestyle and personal empowerment. Nobody gets to tell you *No*—not to anything. All I ask is that you put yourself in the frame of mind of making choices. Be strategic. Ask yourself, *Is this worth its cost?* There will be days and times when it's an easy yes, and there will be others when you recognize that it's not.

Occasionally you will miscalculate. We all do. When that happens, if you're taking good care of yourself *most of the time*, your body will let you know it. And it will also be forgiving as you course correct and move on. With that in mind, I want you to always look at your diet in terms of *choosing*, not *cheating*. Even the most svelte, stunning woman with that je ne sais quoi has an éclair or a baguette sometimes, and she's no less fabulous for it.

Chapter 4

Breakthrough Sleep: Snooze or Lose

At one period in my life, the basement was the dumping ground of our home. It was cold, dark, and airless, filled with containers of unorganized Christmas lights, family mementos, my sons' cast-off childhood toys, framed photos filled with memories, and endless boxes of I-don't-know-what—all gathering dust. This was before Facebook Marketplace, a time when the items collecting in the corners of our lives seemed a little more fixed than they do now. My husband and I had plans to clean it up, to make it a livable space with a nice office, but life always got in the way. As a result, when I needed to work at home, a desk in the corner of that dark, crowded basement became my functional but slightly depressing office.

At the time I was obsessed with the paleo diet. I mean *obsessed*. I love it when history, health advice, and common sense align—and here was something that ticked all three boxes. It was this same obsession with all things paleo that would eventually lead me to learning about bone broth.

In my small suburban clinic, I told all my patients about this diet and how logical it is to the body. The doctor (and, if we're being honest, the overachiever) in me wanted to reach more people. I begged a publisher for a book deal—and I got one. The only problem? I'd never written a book. It would be easy, no? Something I could do on my lunch hours? Once I started writing, I got a clue. I get the chills just thinking about the number of hours I spent in that dark basement, at that small desk, trying to write just a *table of contents*. I knew the work was important. It would be one of the first paleo books on the market. But I was out of my league trying to master an entirely new skill set, see my patients, and take care of my family.

Consequently, this was a time in my life where sleep was almost nonexistent. If you've ever seen *The Queen's Gambit*, where the main character sees the chess pieces move on the ceiling, that was me. The words of my book would keep me up at night. I would see them on the ceiling. I'd be up and down multiple times trying to "catch" them and write things down. I couldn't shut it off. I was a ruminator to my core, constantly replaying and reworking scenarios in my head.

At the same time, I was skimping on sleep night after night and week after week, and I piled on weight. I got wide and thick. I aged *years* in a matter of months. There I was: a doctor, writing about a diet that could help you live a longer, healthier life, and I was slowly killing myself to get the words on the pages. If you passed me in Target back then and looked in my eyes, you would've thought, *she's given up.* Ironically, I was trying harder than ever.

And isn't that exactly how life is? One big ironic mess? My wake-up call came amid a long, grueling stretch where I just flat-out refused to practice what I preached. Adhering to a paleo diet when you refuse to sleep? Like swimming with all your might while you're tied to an anchor. An exercise in futility. It wasn't until I finally stopped struggling, looked at my crisis, crawled into my bed, and decided to make sleep a priority that I finally, slowly started coming back to life.

And that, in a nutshell, is why I've got so many questions about your relationship with sleep.

- Do you sleep enough?
- Do you wish you needed less sleep?
- Do you wake up in the middle of the night?
- Do you have trouble falling asleep?
- Do you wake up rested?
- Do you wake up exhausted?
- Do you want to murder your snoring partner?
- Do you eat in bed?

That's just for starters, because in my experience, *most* people who come to me for help with their own breakthroughs have sleep woes. And many of them fall into one of two categories: Routine Wrecks and Last Priority People.

The Routine Wreck changes it up every night. One night you're asleep on the couch mid-episode of *Bridgerton*. The next night you're up until all hours scrolling Instagram. Some nights you go through your multi-step, multi-product skincare routine, and some nights you find brushing your teeth an insurmountable challenge. Some nights you wear pajamas and other nights you crash still wearing your clothes. In other words, your routine is a wreck. And it's simply a wreck because you don't have one.

If you're a Last Priority Person, you have probably used the phrase, "I'll sleep when I'm dead." When things get busy, sleep is the first thing to fall by the wayside in your life. Deadline for work? Just keep typing. Great new show on Netflix? What's one more episode? Gotta show up at your child's school or the neighborhood picnic with a baked good? Bedtime feels like the right time to bake and decorate those cupcakes by hand. In short, sleep is never your priority.

I get it; it's the one thing we can control. The one thing we feel like we can put on or off our to-do list as necessary. I've met *a lot* of people who feel this way. One of them, a single mom named Laura who'd raised three kids who were just starting out in the world on their own, stays in my mind. She finally had time to put herself first, and what she most wanted to do was drop some weight, get in shape, and feel more energetic. She'd been feeling heavy and low, and she was determined to brighten up from the inside out.

This woman was a dream patient. To jump start her weight loss, she adopted my Bone Broth Diet like a champ. She faithfully followed an intermittent fasting plan. She made time to move her body every day. She was doing everything right, but she wasn't getting results. Instead, she felt sluggish, and the weight wasn't coming off. I had a guess about the root of the problem, and on that hunch, I asked Laura to wear a sleep-tracking device. The data it gave us made it crystal clear what was derailing her progress: she was getting just a few hours of sleep each night (six hours or less most days).

When we talked about it, another important facet of Laura's story came out—the fact that for the first time in twenty-five years, she was home alone at night, and she was struggling to get comfortable with that adjustment. She had a big-screen TV in the bedroom and had gotten in the habit of leaving it on when she went to bed. The sound of people chattering in the background helped her drift off to sleep.

This was a bittersweet revelation. Laura was in an emotional cocoon during a big transition, and she was creating a little comfort for herself. Unfortunately, the same thing that was providing that solace was also producing the sound, heat, and light that were the most likely culprits in keeping her from sleeping soundly. Clearly this was not a moment for me to come into Laura's life like some kind of wellness storm trooper, demanding she give up the one tool she'd found to help her feel better until she was ready to emerge from that cocoon on her own.

Instead we talked about small adjustments. First, she agreed to use a tablet or laptop to drift off, instead of the fifty-inch screen on the wall. Then she agreed to put that device on a timer, so her background noise would shut off after two hours (eventually winnowing down to one hour). She hung an extra layer of curtain over the bedroom window to block out light. And she put a fan beside her bed to help cool the room and create soft ambient noise. Then, according to both her own account and the tracking device, Laura slept. It took about four weeks for her to establish a new rhythm of sleeping and waking, to gently coax her body until she was sleeping seven to eight hours almost every night.

Once she did that, the weight she'd been fighting started to melt off. The next time I saw Laura in person, she looked fabulous—glowing and trim and happy. We both knew she didn't need me anymore because she'd reclaimed her confidence, her figure, and her health.

The thing is that Laura's case is one of millions. The problem of sleep deprivation spilling over into other areas of wellness is so common and so widely overlooked that a lot of us have come to accept it as the natural state of things. Laura's sleep deficit amounted to an hour or two each night, compounded over a period of a few months. Like so many people who suffer from sleep deprivation over long stretches of time, she didn't even know it was happening.

Over the years I've seen much more severe cases—all ultimately corrected by focusing first on this biological need people tend to think is negotiable. We "borrow" or "steal" an hour or two from sleep to do work, spend more time with our families, get in a workout, or just watch that steamy new TV series. But when we make a habit of it, we are borrowing from our own health. Sooner or later, the body always comes collecting on that debt.

Studies tell us that roughly a third of Americans are chronically sleep deprived. That's a *lot* of people who've trained themselves to trudge forward when their bodies are begging for rest. If you're one of that crew, it's time to make a change, and I can help. This is so important because in the hierarchy of lifestyle choices that can wreck your looks, undermine your mental well-being, sap your energy, and make you sick—not getting enough sleep is *number one*.

I know life is busy. Every book deadline causes me to make tough choices about what matters most. During the weeks before my new bone broth products were launching, I felt compelled to stay up all hours tweaking the marketing. And I remember exactly how it felt to lay my head down, start to close my eyes—and then realize my son's soccer uniform wasn't clean. Being a mom may be the ultimate test of stamina, but even in those superhero years when your kids are little, you can only push so far, because . . .

Sleep Always Wins

Ever been so tired that all you can do is think about finding a place to lie down and close your eyes?

Even more than your body demands to be fed, it *demands* sleep. When you don't meet that mandate, your body pushes back. The first signs are subtle—things like drowsiness, difficulty concentrating, irritability, and emotional wobbles where it seems like everything yo-yos between being hysterically funny or hopelessly tragic. In large part, this is because the same hormones that regulate sleep also regulate emotions. Epinephrine, serotonin, and dopamine all play critical roles in both sleep and mood—and when you mess with one, you mess with the balance of the entire system.

Most of us start giving in when those first signs of deprivation become pronounced, but there are times when you've probably pushed past them—maybe for a sick child (or parent), a professional obligation, or because you're traveling and can't get to a bed. Whatever the case, you discovered that the next level of sleep-deprivation symptoms is hard core—things like paranoia, hallucinations, and that disembodied feeling of not being able to put one foot in front of the other.

If you push it even further, the next step—*the last step*—your body will take is simply cutting your consciousness out of the equation. Your mind and body will eventually collaborate to lay you down, even against your will.

It's easy to think that this is only about extremes, that if you're not staying up for days on end there's nothing to worry about. In reality, the damaging effects of sleep deprivation start at a low level—with nothing more than routinely missing out on an hour a night or a few hours each week. The results of that kind of drip-by-drip deprivation may take time to become clear, but they can have a devastating effect on how you look, how you feel, and how well you're able to function.

If you picture your wellness needs like a pyramid, with each level made possible by the stability of the one below, sleep is the foundation. Unless that need is met, you're in survival mode—and your efforts at everything from eating your veggies to taking that Pilates class to doing the daily crossword puzzle suffer for it. That's the thing about foundations: if they're weak, everything you put on top is likely to crumble. Sleep can truly make the difference between dragging yourself through your days, looking and feeling worn and tired, and strutting along like you've got the world on a string.

Am I saying sleep solves all your problems? Afraid not. What I *am* saying is that it's hard to improve anything in your life until you get this one facet of it squared away. Let's look at why this is so important—and then at exactly how you can get your body on a sleep schedule that'll become an easy, welcome part of your lifestyle.

How Much Is Enough?

The ideal amount of sleep is a Goldilocks balance: not too little, and not too much. Unless you're among the tiny portion of the population with a rare genetic mutation that allows you to thrive on short sleep (those lucky ducks!), you need seven to nine hours each night to maintain your good health, good looks, and good life.

Haywire Hormones, Metabolic Mayhem, and Cellular Chaos

Sounds like a horror movie, no? These are all things that happen when you skimp on a good night's rest. Here's what happens when you're operating on a sleep deficit:

Cortisol levels go up. We know cortisol as the "stress hormone," and there are times when it's a friend—like when you're facing an immediate threat and need an extra jolt. Or even when you're mustering the energy to start a new day. But when it's elevated for the long term, this is a hormone that can do a world of damage. It prompts your body to store fat. It makes you crave sugary, fatty foods. It makes it impossible for you to feel relaxed because you're flooded with nervous energy.

Fat cells become imbalanced. It's so easy to think that fat cells are bad cells, but they're hard-working members of your cellular team. The fat cells in your body don't just *hold* your fat; they *manage* it by storing and using energy. They also scrub fatty acids and lipids from your bloodstream—preventing them from causing damage and irritation in other parts of the body. And they play a starring role in regulating appetite. When you don't get enough sleep, these cells sit down on the job and stop playing their crucial role in your metabolic health.

Weight management programs fall apart—even when you're doing everything else right. While you're sleeping, your internal furnace revs up and burns fat. If you don't get enough rest, if you don't cruise through all the sleep cycles like Mother Nature intended, your body responds to the higher metabolic needs you've created with all that awake time by burning fewer calories at night. This can be the beginning of a vicious cycle. If you exercise more and sleep less, it's entirely possible your body's control system will *slow down* your nighttime metabolism to be (ahem) helpful in evening things out.

Over the years I've had many patients come to me in the middle of this complicated situation. They're getting up earlier, working out more, punishing their bodies for results—and not getting them because they're not experiencing that smooth, slow metabolic burn at night.

It ages your face (and the rest of you, too). We all know this from experience. We see it in ourselves and others. We know "You look tired" is never a compliment. Researchers have tried to pin down exactly what's different about the faces of people who haven't slept sufficiently versus those who have, and the symptoms observers note are essentially a what-makes-you-look-old list, among them sagging eyelids, dark circles under eyes, droopy mouths, and pronounced wrinkles. Truth be told, the quickest way to put ten years on your face is to skimp on sleep for a few consecutive days.

It is associated with devastating kinds of illness. Research tells us sleep deprivation is associated with an increased risk for several different cancers, depression and dementia, high blood pressure, diabetes, stroke, and coronary heart disease. There are others, too, but I can't imagine you need a more extensive list than this to convince yourself to make this a priority.

One of the key things to remember about the relationships between all these conditions and sleep is that, for the most part, scientists still don't fully understand the mechanics of them. Many aspects of sleep remain among the great mysteries of physiology. The implications of this for us today are that we have to respect the sleep-wake cycle as a critical factor in our good health. We don't have any hacks or shortcuts to get around meeting that need because we don't understand precisely how the magic happens.

When It's Sleep *or* Exercise

I hope you never have to choose. But who am I kidding? We live in a crazy, busy world, and sometimes I have to make this difficult choice, too. I'm going to make this statement and stand by it: if you absolutely must choose between sleep and exercise, choose sleep. You can't be at peak health without exercise, but without sleep every aspect of physical and mental health is at risk.

Exercise can be cumulative—you can get it to add up over the course of a day by doing a little at a time (we'll talk about this in detail in chapter 5). You can take the stairs at home or at work (or take them twice, or at a trot); you can do lunges while you brush your teeth; you may be able to squeeze in fifteen or twenty minutes of resistance training at lunch or after work. And you can skip a day of exercise without compromising your well-being for that day or the ones to follow.

Not so with sleep. Just one day without it results in decreased blood flow to your brain. The CDC equates the effects of just that seemingly small amount of deprivation with having a blood alcohol level of .10—higher than the level that makes it a crime to drive.

What's more, sleep is best when it's contiguous—those seven to nine hours all in a row. That's because sleep is all about that natural rhythm: from day to night and back again, and from cycle to cycle while you're in it. And while you're sleeping, your trillions of cells are performing their own cycles—cleaning, resting, renewing for another day. Trust me when I say you want and need all of this to happen. We want our cells to flow with energy, not pile up and decay like the stuff in someone's house in an episode of *Hoarders*.

What Sleep Gives

For me, knowing the potentially dire consequences of sleep deprivation is enough to shuffle my priorities until getting enough of it sits at the top of my list. If you prefer the carrot to the stick, though, there are plenty of wonderful things that go *right* in the body when you consistently meet your sleep needs. I guarantee you there is no other lifestyle choice you can make that'll give you more return on less effort than making those seven to nine hours of shut-eye a priority.

These are just a few of the reasons why the hours you sleep are the building blocks of replenishment:

Your cells clean house. Cellular turnover happens in sleep. Picture your cells opening their doors and sweeping out all the dust and debris of the day. This is your body's most important restoration period for nearly every organ and function.

Your muscles repair. As you fall into deep sleep, your pituitary gland releases growth hormone, and the blood flow to your muscles increases. This wash of oxygen, nutrients, and stimulating hormone repairs and replenishes your body. If you've been working out, this is where you get the return on your investment—when those muscles repair, strengthen, and lengthen. If you don't get enough sleep or if your sleep cycle is disturbed, your body misses out on this restorative state.

Your mind makes memories and solves problems. You know that recommendation to "sleep on it" when you're puzzling over a problem or making a big decision? Turns out it's a lot more useful than an excuse to get you to go to bed. Sleep plays a major role in boosting reproduction of the cells involved in brain repair. It sharpens your memories, improves your problem-solving skills, and helps you process and compartmentalize the challenges of the day.

Your bones get strong. This is important for everyone but *especially* important for postmenopausal women. Sleep is essential for maintaining the strength of bones, ligaments, cartilage, and tendons. One study of over one thousand postmenopausal women found that those who slept five hours or less per night had significantly lower bone mineral density compared to women who slept seven hours. In effect, the women who slept less had "older" bones.

Waves wash through your brain. During your deepest sleep stage, cerebrospinal fluid flows in and out of your brain in waves, washing away proteins that are linked to cell damage, inflammation, and Alzheimer's disease. Without that nightly flow, those proteins can build up, making it ever harder for you to get the sleep you need—and ultimately putting you at risk for serious health conditions.

Your body clock resets. Deep in your brain, in the hypothalamus, there's a group of thousands of neurons that serve as your personal master clock. This tiny power center coordinates all the uniquely timed cycles of the body. Nearly every cell, tissue, and organ is impacted by the business it conducts. Sleep is a critical component of these cycles, kicking off the actions of renewing and refreshing you from the inside out.

The Bone Broth–Sleep Connection

When people start adding bone broth to their diets on a regular basis, they typically have high hopes for weight loss, an energy boost, and easing digestive problems. I see all of these things happen every day, and they can be life-changing. The bone broth benefit that shocks a lot of newbies to the lifestyle, though, is the fact that they're sleeping like babies.

In fact, lots of people discover that better sleep is the first benefit they experience from the bone broth lifestyle. There are a number of nutrients in bone broth that can help you sleep more soundly at night and feel more rested in the daytime, but two stand out as superstars.

The first is *glycine*: Bone broth is one of the best dietary sources of this powerful and widely beneficial amino acid. It increases your serotonin levels, which encourages deeper and more restful sleep. It can also help lower your body temperature to help you fall asleep faster. While you're sleeping, glycine keeps working throughout the body on a host of important jobs, from aiding in the detoxification of your cells to improving your blood flow to regulating the secretion of human growth hormone (HGH)—which increases your body's ability to burn fat and sculpt muscle.

The other critical component of bone broth that aids in sleep is *magnesium*. This critical mineral relaxes your muscles and helps to regulate your internal clock. Like glycine, magnesium doesn't stop at sleep support. It is a helper molecule that supports hundreds of reactions in the body, including sending messages through your nervous system, making new proteins from the building blocks of amino acids, and repairing your genes.

What You Can Do

When my sons were little, I made sure they had a healthy, regular sleep schedule. Like all children, they needed routine, predictability, and rest so they could thrive and grow (and like all moms, I needed that hour or two after their bedtime for my own health and sanity!).

One thing I've learned after twenty years of treating patients is that adults need sleep schedules just as much as children do. When someone new enters my care, no matter what the reason, I put sleep in their plan. Sometimes it feels like overkill to spell it out, but time and again I have seen how people who are deeply focused on managing time are willing to sacrifice sleep to get it. Sometimes a friendly reminder that sleep is not a luxury can help prevent a rude awakening down the road.

Of course, there's a catch: Even when we're willing to approach sleep, sometimes it isn't willing to approach us. We get stressed out, overwhelmed, busy, anxious, or sick and throw the whole thing off. There is something you can do about it. You can fake it till you make it in the best possible way. You can mimic Mother Nature's sleep routine for as long as it takes to remind your body how well it thrives when it lives in rhythm.

My favorite way to look at this is in terms of a continuum from daytime to bedtime. Before you read another word, let me be clear that I wouldn't dream of asking you to spend your entire day prepping for night. With the exception of the last hour, everything on this list is something you can do with small adjustments to whatever you're already doing at these times.

That last hour, though, that's the one that can send you off to dreamland relaxed and ready. Give yourself as many of those sixty minutes as you can for your routine.

The Big Picture

Pick a schedule. Human beings are universally wired to sleep at night and be awake during the day. This is the foundation of our *circadian rhythm*—the body's twenty-four-hour clock. Fortunately, that doesn't mean we all have to operate on the exact same timetable. Your individual chronotype is essentially how your clock fits within that day-night continuum. Maybe you're an early bird, or maybe you're a night owl. Maybe you function at 100% on seven hours of sleep each night. Maybe you need an hour or two more to be healthy and happy. You are the expert at choosing your target time. Just remember that you're working within a framework that wants you to sleep in the dark and be awake during daylight.

Whatever times you choose for sleeping, plan to stick to them, within an hour or so, seven days a week—*especially* while you're working on establishing a routine your body will remember and embrace. If you've got a concert, a hot date, or an important early meeting, do what you have to do, but while you're learning to be a "good sleeper," stick with the plan as much as possible.

Morning to Evening

Get outside. Believe it or not, a good night's sleep starts in the morning. Sunlight (even the reduced amount you get on an overcast day) is a trigger for a cascade of physical and chemical reactions in the body—making you feel more awake, amping up your energy level for the day, getting your appetite on track, and even putting the tools you'll need to sleep that night in motion.

In just one of these cause-and-effect chains, the sunlight your eyes perceive kicks up the serotonin levels in your bloodstream, giving you positive energy to start the day. But serotonin is also a precursor for melatonin, our most powerful sleep hormone. The chemical process is complicated, but the upshot is clear: if you get your serotonin in the morning, your body will have an easier time giving you the melatonin you need at night.

Get a move on. Countless studies tell us that exercise—from a ten-minute walk to a full-on weight-training session—helps us get to sleep and stay asleep. We also know that getting that exercise early in the day helps maintain your body's circadian rhythm. Even when you don't have thirty minutes or an hour for a big workout, make time for at least a short walk to help support your sleep schedule.

Three Hours to Bedtime

Close down the kitchen. There are so many health benefits to the simple act of shutting down the kitchen at 7:00 p.m., and this is an important one. When you eat before bed, your body focuses on digesting the food you just consumed instead of on powering down for the night and performing the critical repair work that happens during your sleep cycle.

Anybody who's ever gone to bed too full (and I'm guessing that is all of us) can attest that it's a miserable way to sleep. Your belly roils and grumbles, you may experience acid reflux, and it's tough to get comfortable. Plus you relinquish that great digestive helper—gravity—as soon as your head hits the pillow.

Now I realize the empty-belly approach doesn't work for everyone. I've counseled plenty of people who simply find it easier to get to sleep with a little something in their bellies. If you fall into this category for any reason, you've got options. The first—you know it—is bone broth. It's a late-night soother that will sate hunger *without* putting heavy demands on your digestive system. Next best for an evening snack are proteins that support your body's natural production of serotonin and melatonin. Foods containing the amino acid tryptophan are a direct hit to this bullseye. Small portions of turkey, nuts, seeds, fatty fish, or eggs are all great choices to give you that full feeling without putting your digestive system into overdrive just as you want it to wind down.

Last call for exercise. There's some disagreement among wellness experts about at what point in the day exercise should stop. A 2018 study of studies (research that analyzes and combines results of multiple studies) found that exercise up to one hour before bed did not interfere with participants getting a good night's sleep. If you start a workout anytime during this hour, you'll be able to wrap it up within that window and still have time for a gentle wind down before bed.

If you haven't been able to find time for exercise during the day, this is a great time to do it if you've still got the energy. Even a leisurely stroll around the block is better than a sedentary day!

Evening Alcohol

If you want to see a bunch of marketing and television executives collectively raise their eyebrows, try being the healthcare expert who orders tequila while everybody else at a business dinner is carefully selecting a fine wine.

You can almost hear the question on their minds: *Good gracious, does our naturopathic doc have a drinking problem?*

The short answer is no. I have a healthy relationship with alcohol, just like I do with food. I also like both my foods and drinks to be as clean and gluten-free as possible—and that's what often brings me to choose agave-based tequila or potato-based vodka when I want to enjoy an occasional cocktail.

Why not get that cocktail after dinner instead of pre-appetizer? Because there's no getting around the fact that alcohol before bedtime messes with your sleep cycle in a big way—reducing the REM sleep needed to restore your brain for another day. The work-around for this is not difficult if you still want to occasionally indulge in a drink or two:

- Drink earlier in the evening rather than later.
- Alternate alcoholic beverages with sparkling water to keep hydrated.
- Select dry wines over sweet ones. And when you can, opt for organic options as well.
- Keep in mind that wheat-heavy beer, whiskey, rye, bourbon, and sugary cocktails sit like a bowling ball in your belly—keeping you awake and uncomfortable all night.

Two Hours to Bedtime

Break out the blue-light filters. Talk about your modern problems. Since the beginning of time, people have been getting blue light from the sun. It's an energizing force, suppressing melatonin and helping us feel awake during the day. Eyes are the key to this process, sensing light and messaging the master clock in your brain to dial down the melatonin that makes you sleepy. Other colors across the light spectrum can do this, but blue light is the powerhouse—doing it the most effectively and efficiently.

The problem is that in today's world we *manufacture* blue light in the form of fluorescent and LED lights we can turn on any old time—and those suppress our melatonin, too. If you're making sleep the priority it deserves to be, the *last* thing you need an hour or two before bed is the light from any of your devices suppressing the melatonin that's meant to help soothe you to sleep.

The best way to avoid this problem is avoiding screens during the last two hours before bedtime, but that's not practical for everyone (anyone?). The next best thing is to activate the blue-light filter built into most of your computer, tablet, and phone screens. Look for it under your display settings. You can set it to be on all the time or to just turn on in the evenings. You can also buy inexpensive screen covers that filter blue light.

Lastly, blue-light glasses can help, but since they're all the rage, you have to be a little choosy to find ones that are effective. Look for glasses clearly labeled as blocking 95% or more blue light. If the percentage is less, or if there isn't one listed, there's a good chance those glasses aren't going to make a difference.

One Hour to Bedtime

Recap today; plan tomorrow. We've all experienced that tight-chested, stomach-knotted feeling that happens when you get into bed and start freaking out about what will happen in the morning—what might go wrong, how much has to be done, how it all looks like one giant uphill slog. That struggle is real, but it's also futile and self-defeating. You need your precious sleep, so rather than let it be interrupted by apprehension, beat that stress to the punch.

Here's what I want you to do. Pick up your notebook or planner, and spend just ten minutes with it. Write down something you did during the day that was a positive—anything you feel good about. Great team meeting? Beautiful sunny walk? Productive conversation? Fantastic bone broth–based dinner? Survived must-have-but-dreaded conversation with child, spouse, or boss? Wonderful. Now look to tomorrow and make a to-do list.

There is compelling psychological science behind this step. Studies show we're wired to focus on our most immediate, demanding tasks—often letting other things slip. A written list relieves the pressure to maintain a mental one. A clever set of studies done by researchers at Wake Forest University found that making a plan doesn't just have a positive impact on reaching our goals—it also seems to free up the cognitive resources needed to carry it out. Why? Because knowing the list exists lets your brain focus on one task at a time without fear that some other vitally important task might be neglected or forgotten. Even better, once you've made that list, your brain continues to process its information while you sleep.

Most of all, the outcome I want you to receive for your effort is clearing this path *before* your head hits the pillow, so worries about tomorrow's obligations don't disrupt tonight's sleep.

Choose something that soothes you. I know, there are a lot of demands on your life. You've probably been on the move for twelve to fourteen hours by the time you reach this point. There may be more to do. I'm asking you to seriously consider making this *your hour.* You don't have to sequester in your room or spend it doing only one thing, but for this last hour before you lay your head down, I want you to ask yourself, every day you possibly can, *How do I want to spend this time easing my way toward sleep?*

For me, sometimes this means a cup of tea (passionflower and chamomile can both help you wind down), a bath, or curling up with a book. Sometimes it means listening to music or doing a few breathing exercises. Sometimes it means sitting down with one of my boys to compare notes on the day (and when they were little, it was the bedtime-story hour). And yes, occasionally it means vegging in front of the TV.

The point is, whenever my schedule allows, I make a deliberate choice about how to use this sliver of time in my busy life. The way you spend *your* hour can make getting to sleep either easier or harder, so try to be mindful of whether you're winding up or winding down during it.

Thirty Minutes Before You Want to Be Asleep

Power down. This is the hard part. Here you've finally reached the part of your day where you can scroll to your heart's content or let Netflix numb your brain, and I'm asking you to stop. Here's the thing: there is just way too much evidence that tech input before bedtime interferes with a good night's sleep to ignore it. It's only thirty minutes. You can do it!

Dim the lights. Simulating daylight when the outside world is dark interferes with the body's natural order. Don't worry. I'm not going to tell you to forego all light. This is not the Stone Age. What I ask is that you *dim* the lights. Turn off the big overhead. Use a small table or bedside lamp with the lowest wattage by which you can still comfortably see. Think of candlelight ambiance and you'll land at just the right amount. Give your body a chance to get that melatonin flowing.

Adjust the temperature. Your body's temperature naturally drops while you're sleeping, and you can help this process and sleep more comfortably if you can lower the temperature in your room (65 to 67° is ideal).

Give sleep an assist if needed. I'm not an advocate of taking any kind of sleep aid every day, but research tells us that low levels of melatonin supplements can help us get the sleep we need. If you are trying to establish a sleep routine, if you're having a hard time dialing down your thoughts, or if you just need a little extra reassurance of a good night's sleep, this is the time to take 1 to 3 mg of melatonin.

The Habit Effect

Once you follow a consistent routine every day for about two weeks, your body will start perceiving that sleep rhythm as the way things are done. At the two-month mark (even if a few late nights or disruptions factor in), you'll have created a habit—and pathways in your brain that make your new routine the default pattern of your evenings.

The lifestyle choices you make to prioritize sleep shows the highest level of respect for your body's natural rhythms and needs. And when you love your body, it loves you back. Once you've got this down, you'll look better, feel better, and have more energy to devote to exercise, hobbies, friendships, family, career—in short, all the wonderful, worthwhile things you love.

Sleepy Supplements

We all know you can't just force your way to sleep. A process that's all about winding down until you drift off can't be managed purely on willpower. It's a gentle process—one that the body gets better at when it becomes part of a healthy routine. There are a number of supplements (some of them easily found in foods) that can help:

GABA. GABA is an inhibitory neurotransmitter. What it inhibits is excitement and anxiety, so it's a useful tool to dial down your over-busy brain. It helps you relax, reduces your stress, and even eases pain. GABA naturally occurs in the body, but you can boost your levels of it by eating nuts, fermented foods, shrimp, tea, tomatoes, and cocoa. Another great source of GABA and that relaxing effect is passionflower, either as a supplement or a tea.

Magnesium. Magnesium increases your GABA activity. It also relaxes your muscles and helps to regulate your circadian rhythms. Dark chocolate, nuts, avocados, pumpkin seeds, and bone broth are all rich with this element.

Glycine. You'll encounter glycine a few times in this book (think of it as an old friend), but it deserves a special mention here. This amino acid increases serotonin, which encourages deeper and more restful sleep, and it lowers your body temperature a little bit to help you fall asleep faster. Best way to get this supernutrient? Bone broth, my friends!

Melatonin. We all know this hormone makes us sleepy. But you might not know you can also get melatonin from food. You can raise your levels by eating nuts, eggs, goji berries, and fish.

Vitamin D. Vitamin D does so much good work in the body, and one of its roles is to help regulate your internal clock so your body knows when it's time to sleep. Studies show that people who are low in vitamin D not only sleep less than those with healthy levels, but they also have poorer quality sleep. Vitamin D–rich foods include egg yolks and fatty fish.

Chapter 5

Breakthrough Motion:
Find Your Body Vibe

Here's something you may not know about me, even if you've been following my work for a while: I used to be a competitive bodybuilder. I loved the feeling of strength the sport gave me, not to mention the definition it brought to my shape. I even went to the Arnold Classic, the ultimate weightlifting event, and got to shake hands with Schwarzenegger himself. I was more than a little bit starstruck.

After my all-in bodybuilding phase, I got into yoga, taking classes and doing retreats until I became a certified instructor. And then there were the months I spent studying and practicing Tai Chi, amazed at the calm this ancient exercise, nicknamed "meditation in motion," could help me feel, even when my life was going haywire. I've been a runner, taken dance classes, and dabbled in step workouts, elliptical training, and barre classes. You name it, I've laced up my trainers and given it a go.

And then one day about fifteen years ago, I was walking by a storefront in New Jersey and caught sight of the setup for a class that included barbells, jump ropes, giant boxes, kettlebells, stationary bikes, a great big sled loaded down with weights—and I thought, *Ooh la la, what is THIS?*

The next morning, after dropping my kids off at school, I was sweating my way through my first CrossFit class. It was an amazing full-body workout, and for a while I showed up for those classes as often as five days a week—even sometimes when I didn't really have the time or energy for the effort.

Some of these forms of exercise have held my focus for a few weeks or months, some for years. Many have rotated in and out of my daily routine as I've spent a big chunk of my adult life in pursuit of the perfect workout, the perfect recovery, the perfect balance. *Perfect.* If you're rolling your eyes right now, bless you. You oughta be. The truth is, I learned a long time ago that it's not the perfect workout for my life I'm after; it's the perfect workout for my life *right now.*

My personal history and my experiences guiding thousands of people through body transformations has taught me one thing above all else when it comes to fitness. If you want to be engaged and motivated, if you want to stick to it, and if you want to reap the rewards, you need to *find your body vibe.*

Vibe-Ology

Body vibe is what happens when you discover and engage in activities that light you up, make you feel strong and sexy, and energize your trillions of cells. It's also what happens when you become in tune enough with your needs to intuit what best serves your fitness in the moment: when to grind through that tough routine to the end, when to switch to something less demanding and more fun, or when to bag it for the day and go get some sun.

When you're ready to turn your lifestyle focus to movement, finding ways to get that vibing feeling is the first objective. Try a class on for size. Or a workout app. Or a team sport. There are thousands of ways to move your body, so it's time to *fit the workout to you instead of fitting you to it.*

Choose an activity (there are lots of specific suggestions below), visualize yourself doing it, and then get out there and give it a fair shake. If you're new to regular workouts or it's been a while, this isn't the time to knuckle down or force anything. It's a time to acquaint (or reacquaint) yourself with the exhilaration movement can deliver on demand.

Now, if any of what I'm saying here makes it sound like I go skipping off to the gym every day like Snow White singing in the forest, well—I don't. I have a family I adore. I have a demanding career. And like everybody else, sometimes I just get tired. Some days I do go bounding into the gym, revved and ready. But other times I have to dig deep to put one foot in front of the other and make this happen—even if I'm just cobbling together a short set at home.

In this way, fitness is just like nutrition: what matters is what you do *most of the time*. I give myself a break when I absolutely need it. But the rest of the time, even when life is hectic, I move my body anyway—and I want you to do the same. I'm going to help you create a habit of embracing breakthrough movement, even on those days when it's tough to get rolling.

Here's why I'll push you on this: when it comes down to it, if you truly want to *turn back the clock, reset the scale, and replenish your power*, exercise is essential. Let's talk about the ways exercise does each:

Turn Back the Clock

1. Body composition fact: muscle is lean and fat is lumpy. Working out regularly shapes and strengthens your muscles (especially if you follow my guidelines below), and that's what makes your frame look young and strong. Ever do a double take when you meet someone you expected to be much older than they appear? So often that effect comes straight back to lean muscle. It is the ultimate accessory—hotter and harder earned than any pair of designer jeans could ever be. Whether your goal is je ne sais quoi or revenge body, muscle helps you get there.

2. Exercise gets blood and the oxygen it carries pumping throughout your body, reaching every organ and system, revving you up on a cellular level. That increased blood flow rejuvenates your skin by delivering the nutrients it needs to cleanse, nourish, and renew. If you want to get a youthful glow, movement is the ticket. It's like getting a sun-kissed glow without the sun.

3. Exercise gives you flexibility and balance. So often, it is moments of unsteadiness that make people feel their age. You wobble a little bit when you stand, or you lose your confidence attempting an activity that used to be easy peasy (like jumping up from the floor when you've been playing with the dog). As a matter of fact, one of the simplest tests clinicians use to assess basic fitness is to have patients go from standing to sitting cross-legged on the floor to standing again—observing just how much assistance they need to make that happen. If you can do it without putting your hands on the floor or on your legs, you're probably quite fit. If you've got to get on all fours to make it happen, we need to talk about your fitness. Flexibility and balance don't just belong to children and gymnasts; they are achievable for almost anyone who routinely works out and improves their physicality.

Reset the Scale

1. Finding your body vibe can make losing (or maintaining) weight a painless, even joyful process. When you're doing an activity that you love instead of slogging away at it, you're far more likely to stick to your program and earn the long-term results you want.

2. The muscle you build by working out burns more calories, even while you're sleeping, than fat. When your body is a fat burner, weight loss becomes a more easily achievable next step.

3. Consistently working out swings momentum in your favor. Every time you move your body, you are quite literally moving closer to your weight-loss goals.

Replenish Your Power

1. Power is, at its simplest, the ability to overcome resistance. When you put your body to good use every day, building up endurance and muscle mass, that effort is helping you stock up on your power stores.

2. A critical component of power is being able to fend off disease. Cancer, obesity, Alzheimer's disease, stroke, cardiovascular disease. Exercise helps your body build defenses against them all. Study after study tells us this year after year. If you want to stay healthy, you have to move your body.

3. Exercise powers you up emotionally. There are four major "happy hormone" varieties you've probably heard of: dopamine, endorphins, oxytocin, and serotonin. Exercise is the ultimate hack to getting a wave of them all. Each hormone lifts you in its own special way, and getting them altogether, all at once, is likely to leave you feeling happy, steady, safe, and loving. Being able to tap into all that feel-good energy just by moving your body? That's your matrix of energy making a statement, my friend: *take care of your body in this way, and you will be rewarded.* I also want to be perfectly clear on one point about this benefit: Mother Nature doesn't give a hoot if you can't do a perfect squat, if your yoga poses are awkward and misshapen, if you never learn to dribble that basketball between your legs or make one perfect serve across a tennis court. If your first time taking a walk in three years is just to the mailbox, that's okay, too. The benefits of exercise come from *doing* it, not just doing it well or looking great while you're at it.

Motivation: To Get Started, Juice Your Senses

If you are struggling to move, if you don't have the will or the energy, I want to help you find it. The tools for this are anything that jolts your body and psyche awake.

First, I told you about my crazy resume of exercise attempts. Build out yours. What have you been wanting to try? What are you curious about? What did you like in gym class as a kid that you think you'd still like as an adult? Start there.

Now let's talk about your morning. How does it start? With breakfast? With a treadmill? With the news? With chaos or kids running into your room to wake you up? Checking your phone and email while lying in bed? I've heard from so many patients who start their days in chaos—and then spend hours playing catch up. That's not the fresh start you need!

Instead, every day for a week, I want you to try to reinforce and protect your morning energy. Here's how:

First thing when you wake up, while you're still coming alive, put on a favorite playlist. You can even make it your daily alarm. Music taps into parts of your brain that predate even language—it nudges your emotions and energy levels in ways neither an alarm clock nor a shower can do. Give yourself a minute to acclimate to the sound, get your feet to the floor, and turn that volume up.

Open your curtains or blinds, and open a window. No matter the weather outside, fresh air and natural light connect with your senses on an elemental level, cueing your body that it's *daytime* now, and that means powering up and getting moving.

Light a candle that has a scent you love. Getting your olfactory system engaged in the morning helps you pivot from sleep to wakefulness. This is a new day with new possibilities. It's okay if your attitude is a little slow to catch up to speed. These steps all cue your senses to wake up and get energized: *Feel that breeze! Hear that music! Smell that scent! It's time to be alive.* All-told, this is a three-minute hack that puts your nervous system on blast that a new day has begun.

Next step: A mantra. Tell yourself something good. Say it out loud because the acts of speaking and hearing words have power (more about why this is true coming up in chapter 6). At this point, no more than ten minutes into your morning, you're at a crossroads. What you do next might become part of your daily routine. Consider kicking off your body vibe in this moment when your senses are alert, your mind is focused on the coming day, and you have a window of opportunity to attach an exercise habit to the whole experience.

Fact is that the best way to adopt a new habit is to piggyback it onto one you already have. You turn on the music, open the window, light a candle, say your mantra, brush your teeth. . . . This is the perfect moment to make exercise part of that routine. Why not attach another habit to your new string of morning habits? For example, doing twenty squats while you're standing at the sink. Another great time to add a new habit? In conjunction with a meal. If you take an hour lunch, could you take a walk and climb two flights of stairs for twenty minutes of it?

If you're thinking these things are small potatoes, think again. If you adopted just these two habits, even only on weekdays, by the end of the first week you'd have done one hundred squats and one hundred minutes of steps and stairs. That's an awesome start toward a new routine and a higher level of fitness.

Whatever you decide you want to do, as part of your morning routine and in your larger pursuit of finding your body vibe, consider sticking with it for three weeks before deciding if you want to keep it or move on. That's a fair trial, and it's enough time for your nervous system to create new neural pathways that help these things become a habit.

Here's a bonus tip: If you're trying to extend a fast into the late morning, if you're feeling hangry but not ready to eat heavy, or if you're just having a hard time finding the ideal moment each day to incorporate bone broth into your diet, try making it part of your morning routine. On busy mornings, I put bone broth in my mug and go about my business. It's nice to know my body is getting the nutrients I need to set my day off right—without me having to so much as dirty a plate.

Breakthrough Movement in Practice

In chapter 3, we talked about the basic components of the breakthrough diet—and the fact that there are an infinite number of food combinations you can put on your plate while staying well within the guidelines.

Breakthrough motion operates the same way: basic objectives, groups of major movement types, and endless possibilities for how to build a plan that works perfectly for you.

Here's what I recommend, in three easy pieces.

1. One Hour of Movement Every Day

This isn't the hour that gets you ripped. It is the hour that helps you breathe better, gives you an edge against disease, and reminds you that you are an energetic being who needs to move in order to thrive.

Now don't freak out on me. I didn't say an hour on the treadmill or an hour in the gym. I didn't say *which* hour, or an hour *at once*, or *how* you should spend it. This one hour is the difference between you leading a sedentary life and a moderately active one—and that's an important line. You can break your hour into smaller segments and still benefit from it.

For example, on a busy workday you might spend an early-morning fifteen minutes doing squats, then find three 15-minute intervals later in the day to get moving. Walk the dog, hop on the rowing machine, follow along with a free fitness app—anything that fits with the time you have and matches your body vibe. Even going shopping is better than nothing! On the days you find this most challenging, give yourself credit for every little bit of motion: Grocery shopping? Ten minutes. Laundry folding? Five minutes. Playing with your kids at the park? Fifteen minutes. Housework? Twenty minutes. They all count.

One note to remember: The earlier you can fit some of this movement into your day, the more energetic, healthy momentum you'll carry with you from morning into afternoon and evening. In my own life, I love to squeeze in a little cardio in the morning whenever possible so I can bask in those happy hormones while I go about my business.

2. Resistance Two to Three Times a Week

Resistance is the key to building strength. This fact is built into our genetic code, just as logical and clear as our hinged knees and ball-and-socket shoulders.

I like to think of resistance training in terms of four major categories of movement: Push, Pull, Squat, and Lift. This means lifting weights, using exercise bands, or doing exercises like planks and pushups that use your body weight as resistance. You don't have to go to a gym to make this happen. Yoga, Pilates, bodybuilding, CrossFit training, and body-weight training all incorporate resistance work.

This part of your body vibe isn't about time so much as it's about intensity. It's an opportunity to push yourself, go a little hard, and reap the rewards of those efforts. Resistance training strengthens your muscles and optimizes the hormones you need to maintain lean muscle mass. For the maximum muscle-building benefits, I recommend doing resistance workouts at least twice a week, making sure to enlist an overall workout that includes arm, leg, and core exercises.

Want an easy classic that ticks a lot of boxes? Push-ups. This humble exercise that's been a part of PE classes for as long as gym teachers have had whistles harnesses your body weight to build new muscle. Smart, efficient, and effective—and it counts as *push*, *pull*, AND *lift*. Who doesn't love a three-for-one bargain?

Another great exercise you can do in minutes at home is the wall squat. Stand with your back up against a wall, walk your legs out until your thighs are parallel to the floor, and hold that pose for as long as you can.

Any kind of rowing engages muscles throughout your body in resistance—regardless of whether you're sitting on a rowing machine or perched on the bench of an actual rowboat in the water.

And if you're like me—frequently traveling or struggling to find enough time to get to the gym—exercise bands are the most effective, inexpensive gadget in your arsenal. If you want to use my full exercise-band workout, check it out on my blog at DrKellyann.com.

You can absolutely add resistance training to your routine on your own or with a little help from a YouTube fitness guru, but if you can afford a low-cost consultation with a trainer to help get you started on the right foot, you may find that investment well worth your time and money.

Make sure to allow one day of resistance training rest in between each workout to give your muscles time to recover. Also, if you're new to resistance exercises, take it slowly at first. Start with light weights and do only as many repetitions as you can complete with good form. When your exercises start getting easy, switch to heavier weights and increase your reps.

At the end of every resistance workout I do two things that I highly recommend. First, I walk it off. Even a few minutes of gentle movement at the end of a muscle-building workout will help keep you from being overly sore the next day. Second, I give myself three minutes of utter quiet to be still, to feel the endorphins and serotonin wash over me, to envision my blood circulating through my body, and to feel gratitude for the gift of the workout.

I know doing resistance training takes commitment and sacrifice, but I also know its power. Resistance training makes you strong. It slows your aging. It keeps you from getting fragile and frail. If you get into this one habit, its benefits will outweigh its costs every time.

The Bone Broth Connection

Here's a tiny chemistry lesson: electrolytes are minerals that dissolve in water in your body and produce charged ions. Their presence creates a current that is vital to your body. They help maintain optimal fluid balance, so your cells don't explode or shrivel. They regulate nerve function so critical signals can course through your body. They regulate the pH level in your blood. And electrolytes contract and relax muscle tissue, including your biceps and your beating heart.

Keeping your electrolytes balanced is a very big deal for your health. This is especially important after you work out, when their levels can easily get depleted. But the best source of these vital nutrients is definitely not found in a brightly colored, chemical-ridden, sugar-bomb of a sports drink.

Bone broth is a far healthier source of electrolytes when you need to restore. It is a solid source of hydration, protein, and minerals, like potassium and sodium—and it won't spike your blood sugar or fill you up with preservatives, artificial flavors, or sweeteners. Because of these properties, bone broth is ideal pre-workout or post-workout. Either way it will give you steady energy and help keep your electrolytes balanced.

3. Indulge Your Body Vibe Two Days a Week (or as Often as You Can!)

These are the days I love. This is not about calories in, calories out, it's not about reps or steps; it's about *movement* that feels good from your head to your toes. Think of this time as a weekend for your workout, whether you're able to spend thirty minutes, an hour, or all day. For me, a body vibe day typically comes on the weekend when I have a little more time. You can find me enjoying mine on a bike cruising through Central Park, going hiking with one of my boys, or picking up shells on the beach on a long walk with my dad. Sometimes it's a dance class—which is something that brings me true joy. And sometimes it's a date night or girls' night with actual dancing. I have friends—women of all ages—who spend this time swimming, surfing, rock climbing, Rollerblading, refereeing Saturday morning soccer games, or jogging with their dogs.

When you do any of these things, then yes, you inevitably get your hour in. But more importantly, you tune in—body and mind—and touch base with this side of yourself that should be a source of physical and spiritual joy.

Finding Your Vibe (Personality, Timing, Partners)

During the pandemic, I was one of the legions of people trying to make a productive shift from working out in the gym to doing it at home. It shouldn't have been a big deal for me; I *know* what to do. I know the why, when, and how. I've been working out intensely and regularly since I was nineteen years old. More days than not, I love it—if not at the start of my movement time, then certainly by the end.

So picture me in the summer of 2020, in my apartment, filling up water bottles to use as weights, trudging to my exercise mat—and all the while muttering like a whiny teenager who's been asked to take out the trash, *This SUCKS. Why me? I HATE this.* Pretty sure I was even stomping my feet.

Even if you don't know me, I hope you can gather from what you've read so far that I am, in general, a glass-half-full person. I'm a roll-up-my-sleeves-and-get-it-done person. But this particular scenario was kicking my ass. The whole home-workout thing was so unpleasant for me that there were many days when the pouty, angry side of me won and I just didn't do it. I was honestly blown away by my own cop-out. I mean, *health guru?* Thousands of transformations?

Was I just a pretender?

I was so bummed about all of this, and then I got on the phone with a friend who's a fitness expert and told her how miserable I was. And she laughed out loud.

"Of course you are!" she said. "You're a performer!"

And there was the missing piece. For decades I'd been advising patients to find any workout regimen that clicked for them, but I realized I should have been providing a roadmap. And the first turn you make on your way to finding the activities that suit your body vibe is taking stock of your unique personality. This isn't set-in-stone stuff. It's not rocket science. But it does get at the heart of what drives you, what makes you *want* to move. Consider these examples:

The performer: Yes, that's me. If you ever want to find me in a workout class, look no farther than front and center. I unapologetically draw energy from being in the middle of things. Why was I so unhappy working out at home during a worldwide health crisis (aside from the pall that crisis cast over every one of us)? Because there was zero energy in that room. Just me, my water bottles, and some very heavy thoughts. The minute I took my workouts—both my resistance training and my body vibe time—outside: *voilà*. I was back. Recognizing the root of my troubles even made it easier for me to buck up and use the water-bottle weights when that was my only option.

The wallflower: Are you the last person in and first person out of any crowded room? Introvert much? Is your fitness happy place the farthest corner of a dimly lit, hot yoga class? Or a peaceful hike—just you and your thoughts? Sometimes you like to be on the periphery, sometimes you like to be alone. Zumba? Boot camp? Probably not for you.

The I'll do it if you do it: A lot of people simply enjoy and perform better with a workout buddy. If you need someone to partner up with, to encourage and be encouraged by, it's time to find that pal. If you don't have somebody in mind, try a walking club. There's not a city in America that doesn't have one if you go looking for it.

The competitor: Gotta win at everything? I see you. And yes, I have a little bit of this in me, too. I like to excel. I think it comes from being a small girl in a big family. If this is your vibe, look to an organized activity like a spin class, a fitness boot camp, CrossFit—all classes that will drive you to top your own personal bests (not to mention those of the rest of the class). On more casual days, challenge yourself to hike to the top of something, to swim a certain number of laps, or to master a new skill—all activities that will tap into your deep down love of winning, my friend.

The teammate: I once had a patient who worked in the legal system in a high-stress job. She was raising two young boys, taking care of a little farm with animals and land, and maintaining a flat-out ridiculous schedule. With all that going on, she was barely able to carve out two hours for exercise every week—but she did it anyway. Those hours were inviolate, and heaven help the partner, teacher, babysitter, or child who tried to get between her and that tiny slice of body vibe time. Every Tuesday and Thursday night, this dynamo of a woman strode into her local community center, changed in the locker room with her team, and proceeded to play the most physical, exhausting, sweat-till-you-wilt game of volleyball you can imagine. For her, the draw of this time was rooted in being part of a team. After being an athlete in high school and college, she recognized that team sports were too precious for her to give up just because she had a slew of very adult demands in her life. There is always a team that needs new blood if this is the vibe that appeals to you.

The all-pro. If you love to be coached, awesome. I know quite a few women who do their best physical work one-on-one or in small classes led by bona fide experts. If you've ever been a teacher's pet, or if you're drawn to the exclusive feel of having a pro in your corner, this may be you. Embrace it. Splurge if you can. If not, find an up-and-coming trainer who is affordable. There is always someone in the fitness industry who is brilliant but hasn't made it yet. Get yourself a coach and become that woman with impeccable form in the yoga studio or on the tennis court.

The stand-back-I've-got-this girl. If this is you, you're the opposite of the all-pro. You do not like to be told what to do. You may be a workout free spirit. There's a good chance you've never set foot in a gym or picked up a dumbbell in your life. And you don't have to. What you do need to do is find your body vibe. I'd bet dollars to donuts it's outside, under the sun. Walking, jogging, gardening, jumping rope, Tai Chi in the park, horseback riding? There is a whole world of unscripted but still effective fitness at your doorstep, so go out and see what lights your fire.

A Time to Assess

Before we move on to stamina-care and all that means to me, I want to take you back to that day I took my first CrossFit class and thought I'd found my exercise nirvana. It was brand new then. And it was awesome. This was a class that pushed me and made me stronger—and I was *all in*. Five days a week, baby. I'd drop the kids off, race to the gym, bust my tail in that class, grab a quick shower, race to work, put in a full day, go home, supervise homework, make dinner, play and snuggle with my boys, lay down, and for some reason not be able to sleep.

Can you hazard a guess as to how long I was able to keep that up?

I'll tell you this, I did it for too long. I forgot to ask myself the one question I ask of every woman who comes to me overextended, out of shape, in some stage of adrenal fatigue, and who is looking for answers everywhere except the most obvious place: the superhuman level of effort she is putting in when she is, in fact, merely human. That question is: *At the end of your workout, do you feel exhausted, or do you feel exhilarated?* If you're not getting that good feeling or those walk-on-air endorphins, it's time to take stock.

I kept pushing that five-day-a-week deal until I started seeing a perplexing change in the mirror. My shape was getting square. My face was drawn. My eyes were tired. I was putting in all this effort and it *was not working*. To be crystal clear, this was not the fault of CrossFit. It was the fault of Kellyann, who sometimes has a hard time doing things in moderation, who sometimes needs to take a break.

If this sounds like you, take a day off. Heck, take a week, and think about your body vibe. Try something new. Try resting awhile.

In my CrossFit era, I cut back to two days. And the rest of the week I decided to do whatever the heck I wanted, as long as I was moving. I vowed not to get too into my head about it.

Best. Decision. Ever. I had finally found my body vibe. Now it's your turn!

Chapter 6

Breakthrough Self-Care: Introducing Stamina-Care

C oco Chanel said, "beauty begins the moment you decide to be yourself."

This from a woman who was the expert in "it" factor, who had je ne sais quoi by the bucketful.

If you look around at the women who impress you the most, who have it all together, who carry themselves with grace, beauty, and fabulousness—you'll see it's true. They are authentic and unique in the way they present themselves and in the ways they connect with everyone around them. They're also unapologetic about who they are and what they need.

When I started taking the time and making the commitment to add bone broth to my daily routine, I started saying yes to myself. I started telling myself I was worth it. And that's when I discovered another piece of the je ne sais quoi puzzle: stamina-care.

Say what DKA?

"Self-care" has become a catch-all phrase for a huge basket of products and activities that may do you good—everything from hot baths and cups of cocoa to indulging in wellness retreats and telling people who disrespect you to get lost. It's all about lifestyle choices—choices that can truly impact how you look and feel on every level. The phrase serves an amazing purpose, but in some ways it's become a jack-of-all-trades, master of none. Let's talk about what self-care truly gives you: stamina.

Stamina is just as much a commodity as time. If you go all out and neglect your physical and mental health for long, your efforts will come to a screeching halt when your body has had enough. If you make self-care part of your routines, you'll be able to keep going, meet your goals, and hang on to wellness instead of getting crushed by illness. Which is why I prefer to focus on stamina-care.

I'll tell you this for sure: When it comes to halting aging and weight gain, stamina-care is a non-negotiable must. If you treat yourself like you are less deserving of love and attention than anybody (or everybody) in your life, before long your body will adjust to meet that expectation. You will look and feel like someone who's agreed to play a supporting role in her own world. And you'll crash, plain and simple.

Oddly enough, Chanel's advice aligns perfectly with the words of wisdom I've been hearing from someone else all my life: my hard-working, tell-it-like-it-is father. Over the years, I've asked him for advice on everything. What to do about kids at school who were teasing me for being an early bloomer. Whether I should stay in college after my bachelor's degree or get a job and start earning instead of borrowing. Whether to take a big business risk or stay on a safer track as an employee.

To his eternal credit, my dad never just told me what to do. No matter the problem or question, he'd sit me down and tell me I was going to be okay. He'd tell me he believed in me and my competence and my heart.

"Sweetie, *you have what it takes* to answer that question," he'd say. "You just have to look inside. Just remember to know yourself, be yourself, and love yourself."

Boy did I hear those words a lot. And I'll always be grateful that the person I trusted most to steer me right believed I was capable of taking care of myself.

Taking care of yourself, being yourself: these sound like things we should be doing automatically. But when you're faced with the demands of all the other roles that line up in your life—professional, partner, parent, daughter, friend, neighbor, caregiver, coach, leader—the inner you who needs love and attention to flourish can easily get shoved to the back of the line. Sometimes she's there so long she starts to accept the idea that last place is where she belongs.

And if right now you don't have somebody like my dad telling you they believe in you, hear this: You don't belong in last place.

You've heard the adage, "you cannot pour from an empty cup," right? That's why the four straightforward pillars of stamina-care are just as vital to your emotional health as vitamins and nutrients are to your physical health.

- First is the bare bones that we've just gone over in the last several chapters: nutrition, sleep, and moving your body every day. They're the ground you walk on and the air you breathe—your absolutes. Even if you are a caregiver (and I realize that situation can make it feel like every ounce of energy you save for yourself is being taken away from someone else) you have a solemn duty to protect your own health.
- Second is the stamina-care I think of as *resource management*. This starts with establishing your big priorities—your values—and learning how to align body and soul to stay true to them. How do you maximize your personal strength? How do you protect your energy? How do you ensure there's enough in your tank—not just to get through the day, but to look great, feel strong, and pursue your goals?
- Third is *stress management*. In Part Three, you'll find a chapter dedicated to dealing with the fallout of *chronic* stress, but if you can learn to manage your *acute* stress from moment to moment, you can avoid that downward spiral altogether.

- And last, but just as important, is the stamina-care that takes you to your next level—to vibrant beauty, happy moments, rewarding relationships, creativity. It's the path to your bravest, craziest, loftiest, and most joyful goals. This is where my dad's admonition to love yourself really comes into play.

Champagne Problems?

If you've read my previous work, you may know about the awful day several years ago when I was flying from LA to NYC and my body quit on me. In the moments right before it happened, I felt wobbly and disconnected, and I knew I was in trouble.

And then I passed out.

When I came to, if I hadn't been so sobered by the danger of the situation, I might have laughed at the twin ironies of it. First, the flight attendant asking if there was a doctor on the plane while I lay there at her feet, thinking, *here*! And second, the fact that the nonstop travel I'd been doing around the country—the very thing that had sapped my last shred of energy—was entirely the result of a commitment to reach the widest possible audience with my message about how to become healthier, slimmer, and more youthful.

If anybody should have known better, it was me. This is the work I do! I feel incredibly grateful that people care about what I have to say, and that's a driver that keeps me researching, writing, developing products, and counseling clients—sometimes even when I've been severely depleted. As I rebuilt myself after that day on the plane, I gained a new respect for the value of stamina-care. As dedicated as I've been throughout my adult life to fitness and good nutrition, I'll admit I used to think of that aspect of my well-being as something I'd get around to later, when I had the luxury of more time.

Don't go blowing off stamina-care because you feel like it's a luxury. This isn't about champagne problems; it's about keeping your soul and cells alive and thriving.

To say that I miscalculated that—well, it's a giant understatement. If I'd been restoring and refilling my body instead of continually drawing it down, I never would have gotten to the point where it needed to take the ultimate revenge for my ignorance.

Values Are the Center

When I was in my twenties, two years spent studying at the Paracelsus Clinic in Switzerland gave me a life-changing education in holistic and natural health. There, I spent time with patients who were gravely ill or at the end of their lives, sitting beside their beds, talking with them, holding their hands, and listening as they took stock. Those conversations gave me a glimpse into two of the most powerful end-of-life emotions: regret and gratitude.

People who spent their last days lamenting the chances they didn't take, the places they didn't go, and the relationships they didn't nurture just about broke my heart. Those who spent that time looking back on what they *did* accomplish, where they *did* go, and how well and truly they loved—well, they gave me inspiration for how I wanted to live my own life.

That experience made me recognize how big a role perspective plays in life assessments. Your happiness and satisfaction with your life doesn't come strictly from what happens or doesn't happen. It's shaped by how your life fits with your values and expectations.

The best way to truly know yourself—and steer clear of big regrets—is to get super specific and clear about your values. And then stick to them. If you aren't sure what your values are, then ask yourself these three questions:

1. What do I stand for?
2. What do I want?
3. What is most precious to me?

Here's why: In my career, I've had opportunities to meet some remarkably successful people—movie stars, tech billionaires, business magnates, successful authors, and wellness gurus among them—and *clarity* is something all of them who have staying power have in common. I'm not suggesting they all have the same values as you or me. But they do have great clarity about what's important to them.

Do you have clarity? I believe the first, foundational step in stamina-care is sitting down and determining what values are at your core. If you haven't already done this exercise, it's time.

For me, the list looks like this:

- I stand for integrity, health, and kindness.
- I want to foster wellness, help people transform, and shine as a leader and entrepreneur.
- My family, friends, and joyful moments are most precious to me.

This is a first step I've taken with thousands of patients who've reclaimed their health, beauty, and confidence. It's a critical piece of stamina-care, because when you are defined and systematic about what matters most to you, you can steer every other aspect of your life toward these values. You'll have an easier time saying no when something or someone doesn't align with them. And you'll train your mind and muster your body to strive toward them as well. Plus, you'll discover that tackling the decisions that come through your life every day gets a lot easier.

Neuroscience Hack #1: Utilize Your RAS

There are millions of impressions and bits of information hurtling at you and filtering through you at any given moment. They include everything your senses perceive, all of your body's functions, and those neurochemical messengers we call hormones.

Ever wonder how you process it all? Or why some perceptions rise to your conscious attention while the rest stay just under your radar? You can thank a part of your brain called the reticular activating system (RAS) for doing much of that work. In simplest terms, the RAS, located at the base of the brain, operates filters that determine what, of all the input coming your way, gets sent up to your brain's thought center. It's basically a security guard on the ground floor of your mind, selecting who gets into the room where your attention resides. Everything else fades into the background.

Some of your natural filters save you from having to focus on things that aren't very newsworthy. Things like putting one foot in front of the other, buckling your seatbelt, or smelling coffee brewing. You don't have to think too hard about any of that. But if you trip while you're walking? If you're buckling up in a car that's unfamiliar? If the coffee maker starts to smolder? Any of those changes will snap you to attention. Something new or dangerous will grab you every time.

Other filters can be tied to priorities you give yourself (sometimes inadvertently). Like if you're thinking about cutting your hair short, you'll start noticing people's hairstyles on the street, in the market, or at your kids' school. Short hair is suddenly everywhere.

It's not the haircuts that changed from one day to the next—it's your attention to them. That kind of shift is what can make your RAS a valuable tool for living in sync with your values. It creates the possibility that if you set a *deliberate intention*, you can impact which inputs get through—what you notice and what you filter out.

How do you steer this process? By giving your brain a clear vision. Pin those values on the wall and start thinking about what each one looks like in real life. Visualize each scenario like you'd picture a scene from a movie on a projection screen. I do this every single day. It's kinda my favorite show. I turn my attention inward and see myself where I want to be. The goal is to create an image that's consistently "on your mind."

This is what hypnosis does. This is what personal coaching does. It makes a goal or a change a priority, not just for your to-do list but for your entire being. By approaching it in different ways—writing it down, saying it out loud, picturing it happening—you're activating multiple parts of your brain and getting them in on the job of making that vision a reality.

When you get your RAS filters in line with your values, your body and mind work together to stay true to your intention. When something goes astray from what you envisioned, everything you've got makes the effort to pivot, repair, and push forward—in short, to take whatever action is necessary to get you back on track, heading toward the goal you set for yourself.

Think about the power you can unleash when you put your trillions of cells on notice, when you enlist all your positive energy to get something done.

The Bone Broth Connection

Starting anything new is hard because it takes time and commitment. Embracing the bone broth lifestyle is no different. You need to buy or order bone broth. Make bone broth. Keep bone broth stocked so you have enough to have it every day. The lack of consistent commitment to anything is what often keeps us from hitting our goals.

But taking any first step is part of stamina-care. It's saying to yourself, *I value my health and I value who I want to be, so I'm going to allocate the time and resources I need to get started—and to keep the momentum going.*

I remember nights when I was a young mother, putting my kids to bed and then going out at 9:00 p.m. to get milk or diapers at a twenty-four-hour store. I did that because I wanted them to have everything they needed to thrive. It was my job to take care of them. The same way you mother your kids, mother yourself. Nurture yourself. Make sure you have everything you need to give yourself stamina-care.

Resource Management

Sometime before the year 65 (not 1965 or even 1865, but plain old 0065), Stoic philosopher Seneca wrote, "To be everywhere is to be nowhere."

Talk about hitting the nail on the head. Every one of us who has tried to do and be everything eventually realizes there's a tipping point at which it all goes to hell. Work stops being productive. Parenting stops being effective. Even fun stops being, well, fun. Whether you end up sick, bitter, ineffective, or just exhausted, when you reach that point, you've crossed over from ambition to sheer regret because you took on more than you could manage.

I know beyond any doubt that you are amazingly capable. That sometimes you can push through when the circumstances demand it. But one of the most basic tenets of stamina-care comes down to setting a principle for yourself that goes like this: You wake up every day with a finite amount of energy. Everything you do from dawn to night draws from that pool. You know what each task is going to take. You have to make deliberate choices about where to put your energy. Because if you're not *choosing*, you're giving your power to someone or something else.

Why is this so important? Because if you routinely operate in an energy deficit, you're going to start seeing signs of imbalance—things like inadequate sleep, food cravings, energy crashes, and angry or resentful feelings that seem to come out of left field. You will start to age at hyper-speed. You will put on weight. And you will move away from health and toward illness.

Look, I'm driven. I always have been, and I make no apologies for that. I love and respect women who push themselves to get where they want to be. I equally love and admire the strength of quiet, empathic women and joyful, boisterous women who light up every room they enter. Over the years, people from each of these oh-so-different personality groups have come to me as patients, completely depleted. Why? Because they gave it all away. Their energy, emotions, time, attention to detail, kindness. Sometimes their money. Sometimes their lunch!

Even among the toughest and most empowered women I know, most of us have at least a little of this in us. The tender heart. The empathy. But I'm telling you straight up that your generous, giving nature has to have a counterbalance—and that is the presence of an inner bad bitch who's not afraid to say what she wants, what she needs, and when she's had enough.

Sound like a tough balancing act? It can be, but it's the toughest when it's new to you. When you're setting new parameters in your life, there's always an adjustment period. The people who drain you will test your limits, wondering:

Does she really intend to leave that desk at 4:00 with work still on it?

Is she gonna ignore my email just because she's on vacation?

Does Mom expect me to make my own dinner? And clean it up??

She's going to her room to light candles and sip tea right now? With all this going on?

The answer to all these questions needs to be a resounding *yes.* Yes, every time until your new habits become habitual for the people around you, too.

Look, I know, you're busy. You have musts and needs. It isn't easy to figure out where you can do less. And frankly, sometimes you *can't* do less. But setting a principle of protecting your power will move you steadily toward better stamina-care—even during times when you can't just throw your obligations out the window.

Here are two of my favorite ways to build stamina when you feel plagued by obligations:

1. Stop hosting. No I don't mean stop hosting parties. I mean stop hosting conversations—in person, in texts and group chats, and everywhere else this applies. Stop feeling like you have to be "on" all the time. If you're tired but you need to attend an event, then just attend as a listener. You don't always have to be at the center of attention or talking to be a participant. Protect your energy and your stamina, even when you need to physically be present.

2. Embrace being disliked. Wild, I know. We shiver at the thought that anyone would dislike us. But it's just reality. Everyone is disliked by somebody. And when we accept this, it's easier to make decisions that make us unpopular. It makes it easier to ask for what we want. Start making decisions for yourself and not for other people, and that will protect your stamina.

Neuroscience Hack #2: Flip the Switch on Your Nervous System

In a world full of urgency and demands, it's way too easy to get caught up in feeling as if we're putting out fires *all the time*—even when we're not.

Picture this: you're driving to work and a biker swerves into the road. Your body's reaction is a red alert that comes straight from your sympathetic nervous system—the one that's made to deal with "fight-or-flight" emergencies. In that moment, your heart rate jumps, your circulation system switches its focus from digestion to your muscles, your respiration rate increases, and you get juiced with adrenaline and cortisol—all enabling you to handle an emergency like a boss. Faster than a blink—and faster than you can consciously think—you slam on the brakes and swerve to save the day.

You are powerful and miraculous that way.

Now picture this: you're driving to work and glance at the clock. Thanks to some mystery lag in traffic, you realize you're not going to arrive in time for a client meeting. Be completely honest—does this second event also get your panic response going? Does it keep your system roiling, maybe even through the rest of your morning? If it does (and it does for a *lot* of people), we need to talk. Because being late to a meeting is not a job for your fight-or-flight system. It's a job for its counterpart, the parasympathetic nervous system—the one we call the "rest-and-digest" or "wine-and-dine."

You don't need the cavalry to deal with every crisis.

I know what you're thinking. *It's an* automatic *response, Kellyann. Please don't make me feel bad about that.*

I hear you. I live it, too. Sometimes work pressures, relationship challenges, family drama, financial decisions, personal pressures—and even some of the items left on your to-do list at the end of the day— really can feel as threatening as a monster at your door or a biker in the road.

But about that response: It's not *quite* as automatic as it seems. The fact is, there are multiple factors that play into whether your reactions to a stressor feel like an OMG SOS or more of a when-you-get-a-minute thing. And there's also a massive difference between, say, a two-minute fight-or-flight response and one that knots your stomach, tenses your muscles, and disrupts your body's cortisol balance for the rest of the day. (For much more about cortisol, the damage it can do, and how you can lower it, see chapter 9.)

Among those factors, the biggest are genetics, life experience, and the habits you create. The genetic piece is the one we already considered: do your trillion cells think they're experiencing an emergency?

The experience factor comes down to what you've seen before and how that went. We are wired to get used to occurrences—even extreme ones—with exposure and practice. Think about our first responders and ER teams—could they do their jobs if they reacted to any injury or traumatic situation the way a passing civilian is likely to?

They have to stay cool to be helpful, and experience is what gets them there. (The flip side of this can also be true: if you've had a previous traumatic experience in a similar situation, you may be more likely to have a strong emergency response instead of a measured one.)

The good news is that even when circumstances don't change, your reaction to them can. This is where your habits come in, because with a little practice you can deliberately assess a situation and flip the switch on your nervous system from fight-or-flight to wine-and-dine. It's called downregulation, and with a little practice you can use it to save your body and mind a world of stress, as well as the aging, weight gain, and weakened immunity that come with it.

Here are two ways you can make it happen:

Breathe Better

I'm fascinated by health resources that have stood the test of time. I mean, bone broth? Ancient! I love tools that resonate not just with our minds but right down to our cells. They're the ones that work almost effortlessly *with* the body instead of trying to bend us against our nature.

Think of breathwork—the art and science of deliberate, measured breathing to achieve a result—as the older, simpler version of meditation. It is likely the most underrated, powerful, commonsense tool in every person's stamina-care arsenal. Research tells us it can lower blood pressure, lower heart rate, reduce anxiety, improve brain function, help you sleep, aid your digestion—and much more.

All that just from *breathing* in and out? For free, anytime and anywhere?

Most people's first response is, *I'm* already *breathing, and none of those things are happening.*

It's a fair point, but your body's routine, automatic breaths are shallow, designed by Mother Nature to supply oxygen without taking up any more of your precious energy than necessary. When you get stressed and fight-or-flight kicks in, those breaths become even more shallow and faster. All of this happens on automatic, like a self-driving car on cruise control. But just like in that car, you have the power to tap the brake, grip the wheel, and take back control.

So, when something *feels* like an emergency but you can quickly mentally assess that it's not, take what I like to call a breath break (think of it as the opposite of a smoke break). You can do it anywhere. Take ten slow, methodical, deep breaths. Inhale slowly through your nose, envisioning oxygen going all the way to the bottom of your lungs. Now exhale slowly through your mouth, envisioning all those toxic, panicked feelings exiting your body with your breath.

Your ten deep breaths will serve as an *all clear* for your panic response system, allowing your hormone levels to start to rebalance, your blood to flow more freely, and that flood of oxygen to calm and refresh your body.

One more way to use your breathing to turn off your emergency response is to use what's called a "physiological sigh." Breathe in twice, and then exhale. This pattern—which you've undoubtedly witnessed if you've ever seen a child cry—is one of the fastest ways to get your arousal level back down to everyday business.

Take a Wide View

When your body starts thinking, *Emergency!*, your eyes instantly get ready for a fight. Your pupils dilate and your peripheral vision gets fuzzy. Your field of vision gets more vertical, and you (or at least your eyes) become ready to rumble with anything that comes at you. This is a hyper-alert state—but it's one you can reverse-engineer by *relaxing* your eyes and widening your view back out. Look at the horizon. Look away from whatever is causing you to tense up. See the forest for the trees!

When you do that, your brain gets a signal that says, in essence, *nothing to see here, folks, so move along,* and your whole body can start to relax.

Stamina-Care in Daily Life

The last aspect of stamina-care is the one that incorporates things that you might otherwise put in the self-care department: bubble baths and cocoa—the things you can do every day to take care of yourself, lift yourself up, and nurture your beauty and je ne sais quoi. Some days you have time for a few of these; others maybe just one or two. Here's the goal I want you to set as a minimum:

One Act of Stamina-Care Every Day

You've heard of all the classic ways to take time for yourself. Take a bath, take a walk, read a book, call a friend, get a massage or a pedicure. And believe me, those are all great! Especially if you are short on time.

But I also know stamina is going to come when you take time for yourself and simultaneously do something that excites you. Something that energizes you in a way that you haven't felt in a while. In the last chapter we talked about finding your body vibe. It can take some effort as you try on different movement types to discover what resonates with you! Finding your stamina-care vibe will be a cakewalk by comparison, because any experience you enjoy and get juiced by is the one you should make room for in your life. You can (and should) have a rotation of these, and when one starts to feel tired, choose another.

Do you remember the freedom you imagined adults had when you were a child? Looking at the grown-ups around you and feeling green with envy that they could do *anything.* I mean, they didn't have to go to school, they had the car, the keys, a little money, and they got to *choose* what they did with their time. Or so it seemed. As an adult with a world of responsibilities, you realize that freedom you imagined is quite hard to come by.

But here's the thing: You *do* have the keys. You *do* have choices. And you do *not* have to be rich or live a life of leisure to exercise some of that hard-earned freedom to bring new energy back into your life. What would your six- or eight- or ten-year-old self do with a free hour? I guarantee you it wouldn't be the laundry.

I want you to *take* that free hour (or half hour, or even fifteen minutes if life is *that* demanding right now), and I want you to use it like you stole it.

What this looks like is different for everyone, but I suggest you frame your daily stamina-care breaks by looking for any or all of the following:

What gives you energy?

What gives you novelty?

What gives you connection?

What winds you down?

Now this is your party, and I want you to make it utterly and uniquely yours, but here's a little food for thought as you make your selections:

Getting outdoors may be the most timeless and effective stamina hack in human history. There is nothing that compares to the jolt of energy you get from fresh air and sunlight. Go for a walk, sit in the park, or pick up a city bike and go for a spin. Even if you live in a place where the air is not perfect, or where there aren't as many trees or flowers as there should be, getting outside in the natural air is healing and invigorating to your body.

Think about the difference between how you feel in an air-conditioned room and how you feel sitting outside on a breezy day. That natural air is better for your body. You know it. Your skin knows it. Your lungs, your cells—everything is in on this secret, but sometimes we forget we can use this tool at will.

Did your grandmother used to air out the sheets on a clothesline like mine did? Do you remember how fresh they seemed when they were brought inside? This is airing out your whole person, brightening you up. Even if all you do is sit on your butt and soak up that fresh-air energy, that time outside will lift you up and recharge your battery.

Exercise doses your body with more feel-good hormones than almost anything else you can do—plus it helps you look fabulous. And how great is it to tick two boxes at once? Consider that doing a physical activity you love is a buy-one-get-one for body vibe and stamina-care.

Nurture both your extrovert and introvert. During the COVID-19 era, did you tuck into your shell and not really miss being around people all that much? Or did you find yourself (like I admit I did) feeling an unsettling emptiness as you realized your social interactions power you up more than they drain you down?

A note to my introverts: It's a truly wonderful thing to be able to quietly enjoy your own company. But deep down, you're still a mammal, and we are hardwired to get a rush of good, warm, safe, happy feelings when we have pleasurable interactions with one another. Look around and identify the person or group that gives you your strongest sense of community. Then choose an activity that ties you in with them—at least once a month. If your introverted heart tries to tell you to bail at the last second, go anyway. A little gentle bonding will do you a world of good and it will refresh your stamina in a whole different way from the alone-time activities that feed your soul.

And a note to my extroverts: There is power and peace in shutting down—and you don't have to sit still and meditate to avail yourself of it. You can quiet your mind and recharge with activities that engage on a lower level, like taking a hike on your own, seeing a movie in a theater, or putting on your headphones and making the thing that you are doing *listening*. A new or favorite album, a podcast, an audiobook. Take a break from putting energy out into the world by opening up and letting something new in.

. . .

What does a true respite look like for you?

Cooking? Crafting? Writing? Gardening?

Sitting on your keister in somebody else's garden, just smelling the flowers and sipping your tea?

A good book? A good cup of coffee? Good sex?

Travel? A night in a hotel, savored all by yourself? With room service??

Taking a personal day when you neither have a dentist appointment nor are the least bit sick?

Whatever resonates with you is where you should be looking to give yourself the stamina-care you need. The possibilities are endless, but the upshot is that at some point during every single day I want you to put something wildly, totally about *you* on *your* to-do list. The more you get in the habit of doing this, the more time you'll start to allocate for yourself each day, each week, each month.

What follows will be stamina that carries you through even your most challenging and exhausting days.

PART THREE

Common Problems,
Commonsense
Solutions, and
Healing Recipes

The first job I took after finishing my education was with a family practice, stepping in as the group's nutrition specialist. The plan was for me to expand into other areas of healthcare within the year. Of course, plans change. Within a matter of a few weeks, I had a waiting list as long as my arm for consultations, and the idea of doing anything differently went out the window. The other doctors wanted to know what the heck I was giving away in my exam room.

Here's what I was handing out:

First: my time and attention. I'm a close listener, for sure, but I was equally tuned in to body language, facial expressions, self-deprecating comments—little cues that hint when someone has something to say but is hesitant to open up. And, of course, sometimes I didn't need to guess. Because behind the closed doors of exam rooms, a lot of people who were suffering and needed help let their defenses down and shared their truth.

It didn't take long for someone on the accounting side of the practice to come see me, asking why I was consistently overshooting the ten minutes of face-to-face time that was supposed to be my target with each patient. I had no good response to this, because most of the time my patients and I were just finishing exchanging pleasantries by the ten-minute mark! The fact is, if you want someone to open up and share private health issues with you (and I did), you've got to earn that trust.

Second: my respect. If a patient came to me and said any issue was a problem for her health, I trusted that she was right and took that problem seriously. I was like that handyman who advertises, "No job too small!" Far too many of my patients were dealing with problems that had been dismissed by other practitioners as minor or unimportant. I can't tell you how many times I sat down with women who told me another clinician said their treatable issues were inevitable. They'd been told, "Oh, that's to be expected after you have children." Or when you hit premenopause. Or after you turn forty, fifty, or sixty.

Some days, this made my blood boil. These women had digestive systems that were on the fritz. They were tired. They were stressed. Some were carrying around an extra twenty or forty pounds that just would not budge no matter what they did. Many had acne, eczema, rashes, and allergies. And the common thread uniting these issues was a sense that they'd lost themselves—lost their health, lost control, lost their spark.

Most of us have had that feeling at least once in our lives. You start to feel invisible. You start to suspect your best days are behind you. And you're supposed to *what*? Give up? Carry on suffering with issues that you know for a fact someone else in your circle has overcome?

I think not.

Third: plans of action. The last thing I was sharing in my exam room was practical advice, grounded in my biochemistry, physiology, and nutrition-science background. My patients and I laid out plans that included nutrition, sleep, exercise, stamina-care, and ways to break old habits. We talked about the fact that *of course* they could change the direction of their momentum, could feel better and look better. Equally important, every step we put in those plans was designed to move my patients *closer to health*.

This should always be the norm, but it's not. I had patients who were starving themselves. Women who'd gone to lose-weight-fast clinics for stimulant diet pills. Women who were in uncomfortable and dangerous cycles of binge eating and laxative abuse. I saw women who were physically and mentally ravaged by constant stress, and women who felt such bone-deep fatigue they could barely remember what it was like to have pep in their step. Oh yeah, and women who were practically trapped in their own homes because they couldn't venture more than a hot minute away from the bathroom.

These were problems that absolutely, positively needed to be—and could be—managed.

This part of the book is designed to help you do just that: to deal with the health issues I encountered most often in my decades in clinical practice—the issues women still reach out seeking help and support for to this day. You'll find useful explanations, suggestions, self-diagnostic tools, and especially information about foods (and supplements) that can help move you toward healing. As you read these pages, know that I want you to be free of that belly pain, to lose the weight, to begin each day with great energy, to enjoy great food and great sex, and to walk tall through this world with joy and je ne sais quoi. I believe you can do it and that all the while you can be moving closer to health.

A Word about the Recipes . . .

For years now, I've been on a big-time soup kick. I especially love experimenting with new soups when I'm nesting at home—which I spent a *lot* of time doing during the pandemic. That focus in the kitchen seemed like a natural one to land on since any soup recipe I came up with could incorporate my No. 1 superfood: *bone broth*. When the world got quiet, being a little more creative with that star ingredient gave me something worthwhile to learn about, something I could do right at home.

In these chapters you'll find lots of the new, hearty, and oh-so nourishing soups (and stews) I've come to think of as my "pots of gold." In addition, you'll find recipes for easy-to-make meals, and even desserts, that are brimming with healing nutrients. While I developed these recipes with the health challenges detailed in these chapters in mind, believe me when I tell you *all* of these foods are yummers for anyone, anytime.

I hope you'll find some new favorites among them!

Chapter 7

Go with Your Gut: Keys to Smooth Digestion and Gut Health

I f you hang out with any health professional, here's something you probably know about us already: frequently, our conversations turn to topics that make you say, "Ew!" This, friends, is one of those times. Digestion isn't sexy, but we need to talk about it anyway.

Digestive problems are one of the most common things I've seen in over twenty years of guiding transformations. They show up in so many different forms, and all too often they have the power to torpedo an otherwise good day. Some women are bloated all the time. They come to me practically in tears after some fool asks them how many months pregnant they are. Some people have painful, embarrassing gas. *Most* are constipated, at least some of the time. Others are plagued by urgent bowel movements that come on like an emergency every time. As a result of these problems, we've become a culture of people who can find the bathroom quicker than any exit in a movie theater or airplane. And everyone walks around with Tums in their pockets and purses.

Given the private nature of so many of these problems, it's no wonder that most people suffer in silence. Even as the last-stop doc for many patients, I've often had to pry this information out of them. When this doctor says, "Tell me how you've been feeling," trust me, I want to know it *all.*

If you suffer from digestive issues, it may be a small comfort to learn that this is a problem the rich and famous have, too—all the time. As a nutritionist to the stars, I've seen this impact careers and people at the highest level—people who must keep going no matter what is wrong because there are hundreds of others waiting on their actions. When I consulted with actor, television, and radio host Mario Lopez, for example, he was upfront about how much this has been a part of his life. He often films multiple shows in a day; he makes movies; he's on camera *a lot*. And when your guts say you've got to keep running to the bathroom, that's a huge, inconvenient, embarrassing distraction.

Imagine having an entire film crew standing around tapping their toes, waiting, while you're in the bathroom. Oh yeah, and while you're wearing a meticulously pressed and dressed wardrobe *and a mic*. I've been through this myself, especially when I was new to television and feeling a lot of pressure as I appeared on big national shows. I'd feel my guts clench and think, *This can't be happening. I can't be the one to hold up this show.*

Later, when I was home, I'd think about all the patients I'd seen over the years who came to me dealing with that kind of problem *every time they ate.*

Everything Works Together

Let's talk about the root of digestive problems. All your life you've been told, "You are what you eat." Yes and no. When it comes down to it, we aren't actually what we eat; we are what we digest. And digestion is the ultimate collaborative process in the body. Imagine your body and all its systems are like an orchestra, one featuring trillions of cells that are interconnected players. They work together to foster a living, thriving, healthy, happy you. It's miraculous stuff.

The problem with an orchestra is that when any one player is off, the whole entity feels the impact. It can be something as obvious as a clumsy oaf banging the wrong beat on timpani, as jarring as a squeaky clarinet, or something subtle, like a violin playing a half beat behind—but no matter where the root problem lies, the music takes a hit.

Our bodies work just this way. We get a little off, maybe because we eat something that "doesn't agree" with us—and within minutes or hours, we are in pain. Bloated. Crampy. Constipated. Uncomfortable. The more time that passes with our system out of harmony, the more unnerving the problems get: Exhaustion. Belly fat. Thinning hair. Low (or nonexistent) libido.

At the center of your orchestra is the humble but powerful system we call the "gut." More often than not, when you can't quite put your finger on what's gone wrong—especially when digestive problems are part of what ails you—the gut is both the problem and the solution.

The Gut-Health Snapshot

Most people assume that when we talk about the gut, we're talking about the abdomen or stomach. You know, the anatomical place where a person gets hit if they take a "gut" punch. Actually, though, your gut is your entire digestive tract—from top (mouth) to bottom (well, your bottom). And it's not just a physical place within your body, it is an entire environment—called a "microbiome"—that's home to trillions of bacteria. In fact, your body is made up of more bacterial cells than human cells.

Crazy, eh?!

Now a healthy gut microbiome is an orchestra in its own right—a massive one, comprised of hundreds or even thousands of different bacterial species. These all work together to keep your digestive system running smoothly. They govern digestion and nutrient absorption, vitamin synthesis, bowel regularity, and the development and workings of your immune system.

That's just the beginning of the reach of your gut orchestra. Research is continuing to discover new roles it plays in nearly every facet of health. One of these roles—spoiler alert—involves regulating systems that directly impact every one of the health problems discussed in the coming chapters. What starts with the gut and digestion ultimately influences your weight, your energy level, the strength of your immunity, how you cope with stress, and even your libido. And have you ever looked in the mirror and thought, *Holy crap, is my face falling?* Digestion and gut health, again, directly impact the health and beauty of your skin and hair.

You need a healthy and diverse microbiome to support it all. And the most important ways you influence your gut health concern the lifestyle choices we talked about in Part Two: prioritizing quality sleep, getting exercise, your stamina-care. Most important, you profoundly influence your gut with what you eat.

We're going to take these problems one at a time, but for now let's focus on digestive woes and how you can get rid of them, starting with this simplest of equations: A healthy gut equals smooth digestion.

So, let's talk about what factors may be wrecking yours and how you can get that orchestra back in harmony. Think of it as a two-pronged approach to gut health: nurturing your gut with the right nutrition and identifying and addressing your gut disruptors.

When you accomplish both, your digestive system will self-correct, and the belly pain, bloating, gas, constipation, and diarrhea will fade away. I have seen these simple guidelines improve quality of life for thousands of women—some of whom believed they were lost causes at the outset.

Highway to Health

I used to occasionally visit schools to talk about healthy diet and digestion with children, and one of the exercises that was always part of that talk was asking volunteers to stretch out in a line on the floor to demonstrate just how long the body's intestinal tract actually is. Seeing themselves in a nearly thirty-foot configuration usually did that job pretty effectively.

Adults, though, seem to relate even better with the idea of the digestive system as a highway. If you really want to appreciate the importance of gut health, consider that from the moment you take a bite of food until the last waste that remains of it exits in your body, it is on a trip through the highways and byways of your body. It's constantly moving through passages that are lined with both cells and the "bugs" that make up your gut. And those bugs have to be healthy and nourished for them to be able to help you extract the energy and nutrients from food that drive your body to excellence. If you want to get top-level return on investment for every bite you eat, a healthy gut is what you need to do the job.

So often we talk about food and what it does without considering the trip it takes and whether our bodies are maximizing its potential. Choose to foster a healthy gut and you'll be able to get the best possible nourishment from every meal you eat.

Foods You Can Use

Bone Broth

If you're thinking, *Man, she recommends this for everything*—you're right, I do. I don't know any food that can do more good in the body, truly. When it comes to gut health, though, this is a critical tool for so many reasons. The first star ingredient of bone broth is collagen, which can soothe an inflamed gut and in turn help control digestive upset. Here's a fun fact: You can get collagen in powdered form and in supplement form, but its *greatest* power is unleashed when it's cooked. When you heat collagen slowly for a long period of time, you get gelatin. Why does it matter? Because gelatin increases gastric secretions, and gastric juices are what keeps digestion consistent and regular.

And let's talk about another star ingredient of bone broth: *glutamine*.

Glutamine is the most abundant amino acid in human blood and skeletal muscle—and it's a key nutrient for the gut. Think of glutamine as a painter who comes into your house and patches and primes small holes in your walls that have accumulated from years of wear and tear. When your gut is overrun with bad bacteria, you get little holes in your gut lining. Glutamine can patch those holes. After those repairs, your gut becomes stronger. That's how digestion improves. That's how you get your energy back. That's what helps you lose weight. It's also what can lift brain fog and give you better clarity.

Now your body makes glutamine on its own, and you can also get it from foods like eggs and beef. But there are conditions, like during times of stress, when the body needs more glutamine than your body can make, so you need to supplement. The problem is there isn't much evidence that glutamine supplements work. And many of the foods that supply glutamine are also high in calories and saturated fats—all of which is counterproductive. Enter bone broth, a food that's high in glutamine but also low in calories and saturated fat so you can get the gut-boosting benefits without the negatives.

Need more reasons to love glutamine? Here are a couple of my favorites:

- It both helps you sleep *and* gives you energy because it's so restorative to the body. It's honestly the greatest oxymoron in nutrition. I don't know of anything else does that!
- It allows you to lose body fat while holding on to lean muscle tissue.

That's so rare, and it's part of why people who undertake the bone broth lifestyle get trim without getting stringy-skinny.

Berries

Since humans evolved to be drawn to both colorful and sweet plants for their nutritional value, we're basically biologically programmed to love berries. They are the original seasonal food, and there's something soothing about eating them, even before you consider their nutritional content. They are also high in both water and fiber content, making them excellent tools for getting food moving through your intestines to reduce bloating and bellyache. Berries are also lower-sugar fruits, so they're among the best fruits to eat when trying to lose weight.

Digestive Herbs

Consuming certain herbs to help soothe stomach distress is as old as time and part of every ancient culture's healing toolbox. Ginger, cinnamon, and allspice are "warming" herbs that can soothe a bellyache and facilitate smooth digestion. Turmeric and fennel both help ease bloating. Peppermint in particular is a rock star among digestives. It is an antispasmodic (meaning it can ease stomach cramps), antiviral (meaning it can help rid the body of "bad" bugs), and it has a calming, even numbing, effect.

Prebiotics

Prebiotics are naturally occurring, non-digestible plant fibers that can promote the growth of helpful bacteria in your gut. They act like fertilizer, stimulating the growth and nurturing the health of bacteria in the gut. Here are some of my favorites:

Alliums. Garlic, onions, leeks, shallots, and scallions—there's a reason these are staples in so many cuisines around the world. Besides adding a ton of flavor to our foods, they give our digestive systems a boost.

Apples. Apples are rich in the prebiotic pectin, and they're full of healthy fiber. It's wonderful to have an option in your prebiotic regimen that can bring a little sweetness to your day.

Asparagus. Rich in prebiotic fiber and loaded with antioxidants, asparagus is one of the best tasting, most versatile vegetables that can do this important work for your digestive system.

Jicama. Boy, do I love this one. Easy to prep, fresh taste, great crunch. Even kids like it. My favorite way to enjoy this prebiotic superfood is sliced and dunked in homemade guacamole!

Cooked veggies. If digestive woes are routinely part of your life, make a habit of opting for cooked veggies over raw when you can. When researchers fed mice and humans an assortment of raw and cooked sweet potato, peas, carrots, and beets, the cooked vegetables enhanced gut health. Cooking breaks down some of the fibers in veggies, leaving less work for sensitive digestive systems to do.

Probiotics

Probiotics are different from prebiotics in that they contain live organisms, usually specific strains of bacteria that directly add to the population of healthy microbes in your gut. Fermented foods can also be good sources of probiotics—meaning they do double duty to help support gut health. Among my favorites are:

Coconut kefir. This fermented coconut-water beverage is quickly gaining recognition as a superfood. Rich in probiotics, packed with potassium, electrolytes, and minerals—plus it's delicious and it doesn't have an odor that sends your loved ones running from the kitchen like some items on this list.

Kombucha. This product has been a fad favorite for a while, and I think it's here to stay. Made from black tea that's been fermented, kombucha contains colonies of probiotics. It's also loaded with B vitamins to give you an extra energy boost. And unlike so many fad drinks, it doesn't have a lot of sugar.

Sauerkraut and kimchi. These raw fermented cabbage dishes are filled with probiotics and enzymes that are key for aiding in digestion. They're made through a process called "lacto-fermentation," in which lactic acid that naturally occurs is allowed to ferment. The process holds all the good bacteria in, so your body can use it for better digestion. Look, I know these are stinky foods, but they can also be delicious. Frankly, on the rare occasion when I have digestive upset, I start eating the stuff at breakfast. Love it with eggs!

Yogurt. Yogurt is made by fermenting milk with different bacteria— bacteria that are left in the final product. I don't recommend cow's milk yogurt because that kind of dairy product can be very congestive to the body, but there are tons of excellent alternatives on the market, including coconut, cashew, almond, and oat milk yogurts. It's the fermentation process, not the dairy itself, that makes this effective.

The Gut-Brain Link

Lady Gaga explained a frazzled woman's morning in just six words with her hit song "Just Dance," saying, "Where are my keys, I lost my phone."

How often do you walk into a room and have no idea why you're there? Or misplace your keys and find yourself late and frayed every morning? Digestion plays a role in focus, too. It's called the gut-brain connection. What we put in our gut has a huge impact on focus, mood, and something called "neuroplasticity." Think of neuroplasticity like your car's GPS system. Every time you make a wrong turn, it recalculates. Neuroplasticity gives your brain the ability to change courses and adapt to new surroundings and situations, too. This is what is going to keep the brain youthful and energized!

The gut-brain connection shows up in more ways than one. Have you ever had to "go with your gut" when you had a decision to make? Or felt nausea when you saw spoiled food? Or felt butterflies in your stomach when you were nervous or excited? These are all examples of how the brain and gut send messages to each other all day long, like texting buddies. That's why when you help your gut, you may be helping your brain, too.

The right foods can even tell your brain to kill cravings! I'm going to drop a little science on you so stay with me. Short-chain fatty acids are chemicals made by bacteria in your colon when you eat certain foods, like prebiotics. Researchers are finding that these acids send a message to your brain, which in turn plays a role in appetite regulation.

Hello, nature's appetite suppressant!

One Tool That Makes a World of Difference

Nowhere is what you *don't* eat more important than in gut health (which, of course, impacts every other kind of health you've got!). We're going to talk about specific foods that can damage the gut, but to be perfectly honest, one of the best things you can do to ease chronic belly pain and digestive distress is to frequently give your gut a little quiet time to rest and heal.

Our digestive tracts are designed to handle periods of feast and famine, not constant eating. Shortening your "eating window" by just a few hours each day or doing a mini-fast through most (or all) of one or two days a week will give your GI tract a rest from the hard work of digesting food, allowing it to devote more resources to healing.

I have been using fasting as a tool to promote my own gut health since I was a teenager. You know that amazing feeling you get when you've cleaned your house and can sit back and enjoy that sense of order and calm? That's what even a short fast does for your body: it lets the cleanup crew get in there and detox your systems. If you can incorporate this into your weekly routine, it'll give you a similar sense of accomplishment. I call the cleanses I've designed *Cleanse and Reset*—because that's exactly what they do.

And remember: Bone broth doesn't count as a cheat in intermittent fasting. Use it to help you feel full and productive while that glutamine, gelatin, and other important proteins do their work.

Gut-Health Disruptors

Antibiotics

The use of antibiotics has been shown to decrease the concentration and diversity of beneficial bacteria. When this happens, "bad" bacteria (aka, pathogenic bacteria) can move into your gut and be given the opportunity to flourish. If your doctor says you need to take oral antibiotics, be sure to step up your prebiotic and probiotic game to help your gut recover from the treatment.

Artificial Sweeteners

Foods that contain sorbitol, mannitol, or xylitol—including diet sodas and almost any processed, packaged snack food labeled "sugar free"—all cause diarrhea because they reach the large intestine without being absorbed. If that's not enough, know that they also contribute to weight gain (more on that in chapter 8), bloating, and disruption of your body's insulin sensitivity.

FODMAP Foods

FODMAP is an acronym for fermentable oligosaccharides, disaccharides, monosaccharides, and polyols.

Eh?

Don't worry, you don't have to remember any of those terms. What's important is that some people are especially sensitive to foods that contain these compounds—and many of them don't even know it. Instead, they suffer with symptoms like abdominal pain, gas, diarrhea, constipation, and more—the many miseries of IBS.

High FODMAP foods include some vegetables (including artichokes, asparagus, broccoli, cauliflower, mushrooms, green peas, and onions), some fruits (including apples, cherries, mangoes, peaches, and pears), sweeteners such as honey and high-fructose corn syrup, dairy, and nuts.

If you have chronic digestive issues and a diet high in some of these FODMAP foods, you may feel like a lightbulb went on as you read this. If so, then a low-FODMAP diet is worth trying. However, since it's very restrictive and does limit foods that would otherwise be great for your gut, I recommend consulting with a nutritionist or naturopathic physician (or your general practitioner) who can map out an elimination diet to pinpoint foods that don't sit well with you.

I also recommend keeping a 21-day in-and-out journal. It's simple: write down everything you eat—and also every time you poop or feel any digestive discomfort. Seeing what foods lead to bowel problems is a highly effective tool to help you become a detective of your own body.

Grains and Dairy

Both of these food groups are *major* instigators when it comes to GI problems, including diarrhea, constipation, gas, and bloating. If you are eating healthfully but still having problems, it's time to get rid of these foods in your diet—even if only for the short term. In the long term, once you've allowed your gut to heal and strengthen, you may be able to reintroduce small quantities of one or both of these food groups back into your life. But if they're contributing to your gut issues—and trust me, *they are* for millions of people—you need to bid them adieu in order to let healing begin. My advice is to drop 'em for thirty days. You may be shocked at how much better you feel.

High-Fructose Corn Syrup

Did you know that fructose is one of the biggest causes of diarrhea and other digestive problems? One study of patients with unexplained digestive problems found that three out of four developed symptoms after drinking a fructose solution. This is a good news–bad news situation. The bad news? This stuff is in so many products, you're going to have to be incredibly vigilant to cut it from your diet. It's not just in obvious places like desserts; it's also in sauces and condiments, packaged foods, sodas, and even many juices and breakfast foods are "secret" sources of this diet disruptor.

The good news is that since this product is such a hostile force in the body, your digestive system is all too happy to get rid of it. Research tells us it only takes nine days of laying off the stuff to eliminate it from the body completely.

Sugar

We talked about this at length in chapter 3, but it bears repeating that sugar is disruptive and toxic to every system in the body—and the gut is no exception. What I recommend, just like with dairy and grains, is taking a break from sugar if you have chronic digestive issues. Once your gut has time to heal, you can reintroduce small amounts if you want to.

Your Trigger Foods

Many of the foods we eat today are common gut irritants, which can ultimately lead to food sensitivities, food intolerances, food allergies, and poor health in general. These in turn can lead to skin problems. And most diets lack fiber from a variety of plant-based foods, such as fruits and vegetables. I've shared many of the foods that are the most common (and also the sneakiest) gut disruptors, but only you can tune in and identify what's hurting your own gut. I recommend putting on your detective hat, paring your diet back to the breakthrough nutrition outlined in chapter 3, and then gradually assessing how your body reacts as you add foods back into the mix.

Look, I know cutting out foods or food groups can be a pain in the neck. If this is too much for you, try cutting *back* first and see how you feel. In general, though, I want you to think of these food elimination efforts this way: An unhealthy gut is like an open wound—and every time you consume many of these foods, you are aggravating that wound. You wouldn't walk on a broken leg, and you wouldn't pour hand sanitizer on a fresh cut on your hand. That doesn't mean you'll never walk or use hand sanitizer again, right? Your gut needs you to give it that same kind of protection so it can heal. Lay off the sweets, wheat, and dairy for thirty days, and then you can test which of these fairy-dust foods you can add back into your diet in small quantities without disrupting your gut.

Recognize Success!

One of the questions I hear most often—and one I love to answer—is, *How will I know when my gut health improves?* The changes that happen in the body as your gut heals are gradual, starting in your digestive tract and eventually extending to every system in the body. If you're looking for proof you're making a difference, these are seven of the most important signs:

1. You lose the bloat. That poof-you're-pregnant effect you get when you eat just a few bites of food? That's among the first things to ease when you get your gut healthy.

2. The flat effect. You start waking up mornings with a flatter, more comfortable belly.

3. Healthy stools. How will you know? There is such a thing as a Goldilocks stool: not too hard, not too soft, looking like a curved log. When you start seeing those, give yourself a high five—you're witnessing the result of a healthy digestive process.

4. Skin clarity. Little (and significant) inconsistencies in your skin start to clear up—things like rosacea, acne, and dry patches. You start to get your luster back.

5. Energy boost. When your digestive system doesn't have to work so darned hard just to get nutrients through your body, you have more pep for everything else.

6. Your clothes fit better. The changes brought on by gut health start on the inside, but over time (as short as a few days) they start to become apparent on the outside, too. Even if your weight remains the same, you're likely to see your body "moving the furniture around" as you lose belly fat and puffiness.

7. Food freedom. One of the beautiful ironies of gaining gut health is that once you are successful at it, your digestive system tends to become much more forgiving of even foods that once caused you discomfort. For me, this means occasionally indulging in bread or ice cream. For someone else, it might be wine, cookies, or french fries. Once your gut is healthy, it's better able to cope with anything you eat.

Stomach-Soothing Bone Broth

When your digestive system needs calming, the combination of bone broth and chamomile tea provides a duo of soothing comfort.

PREP TIME: 3 min.
COOK TIME: 10 min.
YIELD: 1 serving

1 cup Chicken Bone Broth (page 272) or store-bought

1 chamomile tea bag

$^1/_2$ teaspoon freshly grated ginger

Handful of spinach, optional

Pinch of ground cayenne, optional

In a small saucepan, add the bone broth, tea bag, and ginger and bring to a boil over high heat. If you are adding spinach, do so now. Cover the pot, turn off the heat, and steep for about 10 minutes. Remove the tea bag and add a pinch of cayenne (if using).

NOTE

Adding greens makes the broth more substantial.

Pot of Gold: Easy-Peasy Minted Pea Soup

Cooked vegetables are easy on the stomach and mint is a great soother, so if you're not sensitive to FODMAPs this is a great dish for any meal. In the springtime you can sometimes find fresh English peas at the farmers' market, so take advantage of this delicate treat when you can. You'll have the task of shelling them, but it can

PREP TIME: 10 min.
COOK TIME: 20 min.
YIELD: 4 to 5 servings

be zen if you can spare a half hour. No time? No worries; I hear you! In this recipe, frozen peas work just as well as fresh. And then there's peppermint—the godmother of tummy tamers. When I was a kid, my mom would make me mint tea with honey when I had a bellyache. There's often great wisdom in home remedies passed down through generations.

2 tablespoons ghee or pasture-raised butter

1 leek (white parts only), sliced

1 garlic clove, minced

1 quart (4 cups) Chicken Bone Broth (page 272) or store-bought

6 cups fresh or frozen and thawed green peas, divided

1 cup fresh peppermint leaves, stems removed, coarsely chopped

$1/_2$ teaspoon Celtic sea or pink Himalayan salt

$1/_4$ teaspoon freshly ground black pepper

Extra-virgin olive oil, for drizzling, optional

Fresh mint leaves, for garnish, optional

In a stockpot over medium heat, melt the ghee. Add the leeks and sauté for 8 to 10 minutes to soften. Add the garlic and cook for another 2 to 3 minutes. Add the bone broth, 5 cups of the peas, and the peppermint leaves. Bring to a boil over high heat, reduce the heat to medium, and simmer for about 10 minutes. Remove from the heat and purée with an immersion blender, food processor, or blender (see Note). Add the salt and pepper. Taste to adjust the seasonings. Add the remaining 1 cup peas and simmer for about 5 minutes to heat through. Drizzle with the olive oil and serve garnished with the mint leaves (if using).

Key ingredients for soothing the digestive system: bone broth, cooked peas, peppermint

NOTE

If you use a blender or food processor, process in batches, covering the top with a clean kitchen towel to avoid getting burned.

Pot of Gold: Carrot-Ginger Soup

Nothing feels right if you're bloated, especially if you can't zip your jeans. This is an anti-bloat soup that will soothe your gut because there aren't any ingredients that cause inflammation or gas. We also left out the onions and garlic because they cause bloating in some people who are sensitive to FODMAPs. The carrots are roasted so they caramelize for a deeper, sweeter flavor, and soothing turmeric, ginger, and cinnamon add warming spice. If you have a problem with intestinal bloating, you'll be making this over and over. And did I mention it's loaded with vitamin A?

PREP TIME: 15 min.

COOK TIME: 25 min.

YIELD: 4 to 5 servings

12 carrots

2 tablespoons avocado oil

2 cups Chicken Bone Broth (page 272) or store-bought, plus more as needed

1 (14 -ounce) can unsweetened full-fat coconut milk

1 (3-inch) piece of ginger, peeled and sliced

2 teaspoons ground turmeric

$1^1/_2$ teaspoons ground cinnamon

$^1/_4$ to $^1/_2$ teaspoon ground cloves, optional

$^1/_2$ teaspoon Celtic sea or pink Himalayan salt

$^1/_2$ teaspoon freshly ground black pepper

Preheat the oven to 400°F. Line a sheet pan with parchment for easy cleanup.

Cut the carrots in half once vertically and then once horizontally, unless they are very thin. Place the carrots on the prepared sheet pan and toss with the oil. Roast 20 to 25 minutes or until tender.

Transfer the carrots to a blender or food processor and add the bone broth, coconut milk, ginger, turmeric, cinnamon, cloves, salt, and pepper. Purée until smooth and creamy (see Notes). If needed, warm the soup on the stovetop over low heat. If you like your soup a little thinner, add more bone broth.

Key ingredients that soothe the digestive system: bone broth, cooked carrot, turmeric, ginger, cinnamon

NOTES

If onions and garlic do not cause bloating or gas for you, you can roast 1 to 2 garlic cloves and $^1/_2$ cup sliced onions with the carrots. Remove the garlic from the oven within the first 5 minutes and onions in 10 minutes.

When using a blender or food processor, process in batches, covering the top with a clean kitchen towel to avoid getting burned.

Pot of Gold: Quick-and-Easy Chicken Soup

Who doesn't love a hearty bowl of chicken soup? This one is a favorite of mine—based on a recipe my friend Lynn Feder shared with me. Lynn lives the bone broth lifestyle so eloquently, preparing gorgeous foods without using sugar, grains, gluten, or dairy—which makes them irritant-free and super easy on the gut. My only adaptation to this classic chicken soup is—can you guess?—using bone broth. This simple change allows me to get this dish on the table in about half the time. It also ensures you're getting all the minerals, collagen, and health benefits of bone broth rather than plain stock.

PREP TIME: 20 min.
COOK TIME: 40 min.
YIELD: 8 to 10 servings

3 quarts (12 cups) Chicken Bone Broth (page 272) or store-bought

$^3/_4$ pound skinless, bone-in chicken breasts

$^3/_4$ pound skinless, bone-in chicken thighs or drumsticks

4 carrots, sliced into coins

4 celery stalks, sliced

2 leeks (white parts only), sliced, or 1 small to medium onion, diced

$^3/_4$ cup parsley leaves, stems discarded, chopped

1 teaspoon ground turmeric or 1 (1$^1/_2$-inch) piece of fresh turmeric, peeled but not sliced

1 (1-inch) piece fresh ginger, peeled but not sliced

2 teaspoons Celtic sea or pink Himalayan salt

$^1/_2$ to 1 teaspoon freshly ground black pepper

Pour the bone broth into a large stockpot and bring to a boil over high heat. Add the chicken, bring to a slow simmer, and immediately reduce the heat to medium-low or low. Do not boil the chicken (see Notes). After about 15 minutes of simmering, use a fine-mesh sieve to remove any foam that has floated to the top. (This is protein from the chicken; removing it keeps the broth clear, but this step is optional.)

Add the carrots, celery, leeks, parsley, turmeric, and ginger. Cover the pot and simmer over low heat for about 20 minutes or until the vegetables have softened.

Remove the chicken, discard the bones, and shred the meat with two forks. Return the chicken to the pot. Stir in the salt and pepper. Taste to adjust the seasonings and serve.

Key ingredients that aid digestion: bone broth, leeks, parsley, turmeric, ginger

NOTES

Don't boil the chicken because it will toughen the meat. Always maintain a gentle simmer, which ranges between 185 and 205°F.

You can add zoodles, $^1/_2$ cup brown rice pasta, or $^1/_2$ cup rice per serving for a heartier variation if you choose.

Pot of Gold: Cucumber-Melon Gazpacho

This gazpacho is a welcome reprieve on sweltering days. Enjoy a cup as a first course or have a
bowl for lunch. The soup is filled with tummy-
soothing ingredients that will gently calm your
digestive system. I make chilled soups when it's
hot because they are so refreshing, quick, and
easy to prepare. . . . Just put all the ingredients
in a blender or food processor, turn it on, and the soup is ready. No hot kitchen!

PREP TIME: 15 min.
YIELD: 4 servings

2 cups Chicken Bone Broth (page 272; see Notes) or store-bought

$^1/_4$ cup coarsely chopped onion, optional (see Notes)

1 small garlic clove, coarsely chopped, optional (see Notes)

1 English cucumber (seeds removed if large), coarsely chopped

$^1/_2$ cantaloupe or honeydew melon, coarsely chopped (about 3 to 4 cups)

$^1/_2$ avocado, coarsely chopped

3 to 4 tablespoons freshly squeezed lemon or lime juice

1 teaspoon grated peeled fresh ginger

$^1/_4$ cup loosely packed fresh peppermint leaves (stems removed)

$1^1/_2$ teaspoons Celtic sea or pink Himalayan salt

$^1/_2$ teaspoon freshly ground black pepper

Fresh mint, for serving, optional

In a blender or food processor, add the bone broth, onion, garlic, and cucumber.
Purée until smooth. Pour the mixture into a large bowl and set aside.

To the blender, add the melon, avocado, lemon juice, ginger, and peppermint leaves
and purée until smooth. Pour the mixture into the large bowl with the broth mixture, stirring to combine. Add the salt and pepper and stir well. Cover and refrigerate for 2 hours.

Serve chilled and garnished with the mint (if using).

*Key ingredients to soothe your digestive system: bone broth, cucumbers, melon, pep-
permint, ginger*

NOTES

If you enjoy your gazpacho thinner, add more bone broth.

If you're sensitive to onions or garlic, omit them from the recipe.

If you like spice, add $\frac{1}{4}$ to $\frac{1}{2}$ chopped jalapeño. Keep as many seeds as desired.

Sautéed Cod with Fresh Fennel

Fennel is a member of the carrot family, although the bulb grows above ground. It has stalks, similar to celery, and is covered with delicate fronds that look much like dill. Fennel has a delicate, almost sweet flavor that mellows when cooked and is often served with fish. In many cuisines, fennel is served after a meal to aid digestion. Fennel helps with digestion by reducing inflammation in the intestines and decreasing bacteria that cause bloating and gas.

PREP TIME: 20 min.
COOK TIME: 20 min.
YIELD: 4 servings

5 tablespoons ghee (or a combination of ghee and avocado oil), divided

1 pound fresh fennel (about 2 to 3 medium bulbs), stalks removed and bulbs cut in half vertically and thinly sliced, reserving the fronds for garnish (see Notes)

$1^1/_2$ teaspoons Celtic sea or pink Himalayan salt, divided

4 (5- to 6-ounce) cod loins, thoroughly dried (see Notes)

$^1/_4$ teaspoon freshly ground black pepper

Juice of 1 lemon (about 2 to 3 tablespoons)

$^1/_2$ cup fresh parsley leaves, stems discarded, coarsely chopped

Lemon wedges, for serving, optional

In a medium sauté pan, heat 3 tablespoons of the ghee over medium heat. Add the fennel and toss to coat with oil. Cook 10 to 15 minutes, stirring occasionally, until the fennel caramelizes. If you want it more tender, add 1 to 2 tablespoons water, cover, and steam for 1 to 2 minutes. Add $^1/_2$ teaspoon of the salt and the fennel fronds (if using).

Meanwhile, melt the remaining 2 tablespoons ghee in a medium sauté pan over medium-high heat. When the pan is hot, add the cod, being sure not to crowd the fish. Season the fish with the remaining 1 teaspoon salt and the pepper. Cook 3 to 5 minutes, turn the fish, and cook another 2 to 4 minutes or until golden (see Notes). Remove the fish from skillet to a platter. Add the lemon juice to the pan to deglaze it and simmer for 1 to 2 minutes. Add the parsley and then pour over fish. Serve immediately with the fennel on the side and the lemon wedges (if using). Garnish with fennel fronds, if desired.

Key ingredients to aid digestion: fennel

NOTES

Small fennel bulbs are more tender than larger ones. Look for fennel with the bulb about the size of a tennis ball. The stalks are usually discarded because they are tough, but I've found they soften considerably when cooked. Use a sharp chef's knife or a mandolin to thinly slice the fennel.

By thoroughly drying the cod you prevent it from steaming so you can get a nice golden sear.

Cod loins are cut from the thickest part at the top of the whole fillet and are usually skinless and boneless. They are typically about $1/_2$-inch thick. You can also use cod fillets, which are thinner and come from the back, closer to the tail of the fillet. The cook time will vary based on the thickness of the fish. The fish is done when it easily flakes with a fork and the center is opaque or when the internal temperature reaches 145°F.

Chapter 8

Slim-Gestion:
Lose Weight and Keep It Off

Diets come and go, but wellness is a long game. If you make wellness your aim, reaching your optimal weight becomes a logical, manageable next step—rather than a seemingly impossible, potentially painful leap. Trust me when I say that I know my stuff in this area. I've spent much of my career creating and implementing plans designed not only to take pounds off my patients but to do it healthfully. Hundreds of thousands of patients, concierge clients, readers, and product customers can attest that my holy trinity of goals includes nurturing their good health, tackling weight loss, and improving self-esteem. Truth is, when you try to separate these aspects of well-being, there's always a barrier to the ultimate outcome: meaningful, joyful transformation.

Back when I was starting out in my first medical practice job, a majority of my patients shared the common health concern of wanting to shed weight. They were feeling heavy on their feet, and that was weighing heavy on their minds. Most had biometrics that reflected those feelings: high blood pressure, high blood sugar, and unhealthy cholesterol ratios.

So many of these women had been told that since they didn't meet the clinical definition of obesity (or in some cases, even though they *did* meet it), their weight was of no significant medical concern. Some were even made to feel as if their requests for help were somehow frivolous.

Let's get one thing clear: There is *nothing* frivolous about the desire to get in shape. And if you're here for weight-loss guidance, I am here to help. More times than I can count, I have seen firsthand how losing twenty or thirty pounds can be the cornerstone of crucial shifts. I've seen women use that one giant step to regain their overall health, their confidence—and the je ne sais quoi they may have thought was gone forever. It plays out in so many ways: women who walk tall again, women who smile at me for the first time, women who show up at the office holding hands with a partner they barely glanced at when their journey started.

Is getting to your optimal weight the key to a lifetime of happiness? Nah. But it *does* feel fantastic, and it *can* be a catalyst for happy changes. Think of it this way: Your body is like your business. You grew it, nourished it, pampered it, or neglected it. You've directed its energy into beautiful and even miraculous things. It has given you pain, yes, but it's also given you joy. (P.S.: We're going to talk about sex in chapter 9.)

When you reach a certain age and the pounds start piling on—or you stop taking good care of yourself, or you stop seeing anything beautiful in the mirror—well, let's call it a takeover. Weight takes over. Fatigue takes over. Low self-esteem takes over. And one day you realize you're moving around in a body that doesn't even feel like your own anymore. When you take back control of this precious thing that got away from you—your body, your health—well, there's not much that feels better in this world than reinstating yourself as CEO of your own life.

The feeling of being in control, of looking the way you want to look, and being strong from the inside out—it's beyond satisfying. It's the ultimate fresh start.

So, let's talk about what it's going to take to make this happen. In chapter 3, I shared the foundation of every diet I've ever written: happy plates composed mostly of lean and clean proteins, fibrous vegetables, and healthy fats. But it's extra important to delve into the details when you're focused on seeing results on the scale. Toward that end, we're now going to tackle four key topics:

Gut health (in the context of weight loss, I call it "slim-gestion")

Intermittent fasting

Emotional-eating management

What's your fairy dust: making 80/20 work for you

Slim-Gestion \slim-jes-chuhn\ noun: the power to heal your gut and lose weight

Okay, so that definition isn't approved by Webster's yet, but it's only a matter of time, in my humble opinion. The point of it, above all, is this: any diet method that does not include fostering gut health is likely to end up, well, doomed. Having a healthy gut is truly one of the biggest and most powerful secrets to weight loss. There is a strong correlation between your weight and gut health.

One of my most vivid memories is the day I first learned about this connection. I was prepping for a segment on Good Morning America while another medical expert was prepping with a different producer. They were digging into cutting-edge research about the role of gut bacteria in obesity. The minute my segment ended, I practically ran off the set and dove into the study. Yes, I am a nutrition nerd to my core—and this study was a game changer.

For the research in question, scientists recruited pairs of human twins in which one was lean and the other was obese. They transferred gut bacteria from these participants into genetically identical mice that had been raised in the same germ-free environment. Sound a little

Frankenstein-ish? I thought so, too, but what happened next changed my world. The mice in both groups proceeded to eat the same diet in equal amounts. The reasonable expectation might have been that the mice would remain identical, but that's not what happened. Instead, the mice with bacteria from an obese twin grew heavier and amassed more body fat than the mice with microbes from a thin twin.

Same animals, same environment, same exact calories in, and then—completely different weight trends. What it means for you and me and millions of other people boils down to this: you could be doing everything right and still not see the scale move.

In order to healthfully, permanently lose weight, we've got to get your gut healthy.

This starts with eating, not with abstaining. In chapter 3, I laid out nutrition guidance that emphasizes bone broth, protein, fibrous vegetables, and healthy fats. If you do nothing but adopt that plan, your gut will thank you by getting healthier—and your body will thank you by getting leaner. If you incorporate my gut-healing advice from chapter 7—particularly adding pre- or probiotics to your diet—even better. You'll be on your way.

When you heal your gut, everything about weight loss gets easier—your digestion is smoother, your body is more efficient at absorbing nutrients, your cravings will ease, and, when you occasionally indulge in off-the-plan and way-way-off-the-plan foods, your body will be more inclined to stay strong and healthy.

Intermittent Fasting

Intermittent fasting is one of the keys to any healthy nutrition plan as it gives your gut time to heal. And when you want to lose weight, it is one of the most effective resources in your toolbox. Two of the best ways to do this are to choose a twenty-four-hour fast once or twice a week or to shorten your eating "window" to ten hours or less each day. These fasting periods give your body a chance to rest, restore, digest, and utilize every nutrient it's been given, and to burn fat deposits to replace the energy from sugar that you're not giving it.

For many of my patients, fasting is both the most daunting and the most effective step they take in a weight-loss regimen. Before undertaking this, they worry that it'll be too hard. But they realize after they try it that the body kind of likes being empty. Even when I'm not actively looking to manage my weight, there are days when I wake up feeling overfull from the night before and choose to do a 1-day fast—because it feels like a true reset for body and mind.

Remember that bone broth can be your fasting support system. You can indulge in it multiple times during the day *without breaking your fast.* Many of my patients keep packets of bone broth powder in their bag on fasting days—so they can just add water and get an extra boost of protein, minerals, and collagen anytime they need it. Some brands, including my own, make these in great flavors. My personal favorite is my Thai Lemongrass packets—a flavor I developed with my own fasting days in mind.

Drifting Away? Let Bone Broth Be Your Anchor

Whether you're looking to lose weight or maintain, the time will come when you drift (or paddle your heart out) away from the lifestyle you aspire to live. It happens to all of us. Whether you get just a bit off course or go all out with decadent eating, whether it's for a day or for a month (or more), setbacks come part and parcel with being beautifully human. You are a vibrant, energetic, emotional being, not a robot. You make choices in each moment.

What matters when this happens isn't the moment that's already passed. It's the next moment, and the one after that. One of the things I've tried to do in this book is to be open about how often I have done this myself—and how often it happens even to the women who walk through life with beauty and breathtaking je ne sais quoi. They make mistakes, I make mistakes, you make mistakes—we're all sisters in that. And most of us are also sisters in our shared tendency to be hard on ourselves.

I want to help you get back on track. And that starts with choosing to move on from the self-loathing, move on from the eating regret, move on from any and all extreme thinking about how to undo damage. Say to yourself, "I ate what I ate. I will get back on track at my next meal."

Enter bone broth: Let bone broth be your anchor. Let one cup of bone broth get you back on track. It's your reset. Here's your reminder that:

One bad bite does not equal a bad meal.

One bad meal does not equal a bad day.

One bad day does not equal a bad week.

One bad week does not equal a bad month.

One bad month does not equal a bad year.

What this comes down to, friends, is never giving up the fight. You're never off the track if you don't want to be.

Emotional-Eating Management

When I worked in a small-town medical practice, *most* of my patients reported overeating (or eating foods they knew were terrible for them) when they were stressed. You name the stressor, and I guarantee you that right this minute someone is seeking solace for it in a bag of chips, a gallon of ice cream, a box of cookies, or a pitcher of margaritas.

Here's what I want you to know about emotional eating: it can be tied to *any* emotion—not just stress. We eat when we're happy; we eat when we're sad; we eat when we're tired, when we're wired, when we're lonely. One of the most important ways to become truly effective at managing your weight is to learn how to put a pin in eating that was not part of your plan for the meal, the day, the week, or longer.

Just like how you count to ten before you discipline your kid for doing something stupid, or how you take that deeeep breath before you respond to that nosy neighbor's insinuation about your partner coming home late or that the aforementioned child is somehow naughty at heart, sometimes you need to buy a tiny wedge of time in which to think before you take a potentially regrettable action. In this case, it's not blurting out words you can never take back, it's eating something you neither really want nor need because it is there, you are bored, you have a habit—any reason that has nothing to do with being hungry.

Taking that beat to *think* about whether you *want* to eat the food in question is what makes you the CEO of your health and your diet. *Choose* to eat or *choose* not to eat—but don't just mindlessly consume.

What's Your Fairy Dust? Making 80/20 Work for You

Directly tied to emotional eating is the concept I call fairy-dust foods. These are the things that fall outside (sometimes *waayy* outside) the nutrition plan outlined in chapter 3. Why can't we just stay on restriction indefinitely? Because it doesn't work. Never. We crave rewards. We crave variety. We crave experiences. And sometimes our rewards and varied experiences are inevitably going to take us outside of the lean-protein, fibrous-veggie, and healthy-fat paradigm.

And that is completely fine—*even* when you are actively working to lose weight. The way I want you to handle the fairy-dust issue is in the spirit of Marie Kondo and her methods for tidying up. I mean, who among us didn't march into the closet in search of the distinction between what "sparks joy" and what we might choose to let go? What if we apply Kondo's simple principle to everything we eat—not just while it's sitting on our plate, but while we're deciding what to put there.

Consider making a list of the foods that really spark joy in your life.

Get specific, so rather than, say, cookies, how about a chocolate chip cookie from Levain Bakery in NYC. Instead of just pasta, how about Mom's homemade gnocchi? In most cases, the foods on your list will be truly special foods, occasional in every sense of the word—and they probably do spark joy. They're tied up in the rituals, memories, and pleasurable moments of your life—and there's no earthly reason for you to give these up.

I ask you to do this exercise because most of the time when we fall out of healthy eating, it isn't even for something we love. It's the everyday crap lying around in the cupboard, on the counter, or left over on our kids' plates that inevitably leaves us with feelings of angst, regret, and shame—because deep down, we know we aren't getting our "money's worth" from these splurges. They aren't bringing us joy. Consider a hundred tortilla chips (with queso!) mindlessly noshed during a football game. Or six lackluster store-bought cookies at a barbecue. Or nine random pieces of candy from a bowl at work. There's a good chance none of this food brought joy. In the moment it might deliver a dopamine hit, but that's not true joy.

It's okay to eat what you love. But if you don't love it, let it go.

This is why I always advise that you *let the magic of the 80/20 rule work for you*. Adopting this lifestyle means you can eat non-diet foods 20% of the time, while sticking to the basic diet template 80% of the time. This way of living lets you enjoy life without gaining back those pounds and wrinkles. This design gives you plenty of room for "personal play"—for doing things your way so you don't feel deprived. For instance, you *can* indulge in a glass (or two) of wine at book club or when out to dinner with a friend. You *can* order waffles when out to breakfast with your family once a month. And you *can* keep your weight right where you want it. That's because when you eat right 80% of the time, your body is so vibrant and healthy that it can easily handle a little sin once in a while.

Foods That Make You Go, *Hmmm*

Yes, I did indeed just say you can have anything you want 20% of the time. And I meant it. But I want you to always be aware of the foods that wrecked your gut health in the first place. You can have them sometimes; I have them sometimes. But because they have the potential to derail every one of the steps you took to achieve your healthy, gorgeous transformation, picture them with a "buyer beware" tag. Not for everyday use. Handle with care.

You get the idea.

For a lot of people, consuming these foods now and again is not a deal breaker. Even for me and my long-term nemesis: gluten. I can have a sandwich or a slice of cake if I really want one. Occasionally.

Gluten

More than 80% of my patients have a bad reaction to foods containing gluten. Of all the foods people eliminate on the bone broth plan, this is the one that's most likely to cause trouble when it's reintroduced. I know this seems counterintuitive. I mean, bread? Beer? Cake? Are these not the foods that let us know God loves us? I know it can feel unfair, but for many, many people, the gluten in these foods brings far more misery than joy because it upsets the gut and causes abdominal pain, diarrhea, bloating, fatigue, and even depression. So be very wary if you add gluten-containing foods back into your diet! To keep these foods in mind, remember the acronym BROWS. It stands for barley, rye, oats (which are okay only if they're specifically labeled as "gluten-free"), wheat, and spelt.

Speaking of Gluten, How About Those Other Carb-y Snacks . . .

You know those sneaky little guys that practically jump into your hands when you open the pantry. A few crackers here, a few chips there. A couple cookies. What happens *between* meals is often the most difficult to manage for people who are actively working to lose weight. There are two main reasons to push back on this kind of mindless eating. First, because it'll quickly derail all the great work you're doing to heal your gut. If you've got to indulge in these foods, do it once a week (even if it's a larger portion) rather than a little bit every day. Second, the breakthrough plan is designed to get your body burning fat instead of sugar. But all the carb snacks quickly turn to sugars in your digestive system, and they directly interfere with the process of your body working more efficiently.

Dairy

Dairy is a big cause of digestive problems, and many of my patients discover that drinking milk or eating cheese leads to headaches, skin breakouts, or sinus problems. So often, though, people don't make the connection between these foods and their symptoms. Over the years, I've had patients with unbridled fatigue, psoriasis, eczema, menstrual problems, constant congestion—the list goes on and on—and we've discovered through a process of elimination that dairy is the root of their troubles.

If you are actively seeking to lose weight or if you're in the first month of choosing foods to heal your gut, I highly recommend staying off dairy completely. The rest of the time, though, I've found that some cheeses tend to be better tolerated than others. If you're ready to reintroduce cheese, try Manchego (a sheep's milk cheese with smaller molecules than cow's milk cheese), mozzarella, Parmesan, and pasture-raised butter.

Sweets

If you adopt the breakthrough nutrition plan, you will get your sugar cravings under control—so it's okay to give your sweet tooth a little thrill now and then. Honey, molasses, maple syrup, coconut sugar, and stevia are all okay in limited amounts (although it's smart to stay away from table sugar as much as you can, because it's poison to your cells). But don't overdo sweet foods, or you'll be inviting that sugar demon right back into your life.

Artificial Sweeteners

The pink, yellow, and blue packets are all a no-go for me because your body registers them just like sugar and they're loaded with chemicals. If you're craving sweet flavor, stevia, date juice, coconut sugar, and monk-fruit sweetener are better options.

Of course, one of the places we're most likely to encounter artificial sweeteners is in diet soda. We can all do better than having this product in our diets. Are you familiar with the term *diet soda belly*? Most nutritionists are. And did you know that people who drink diet soda tend to have more belly fat than people who don't? A study published in the *Journal of the American Geriatrics Society* found that people who drank diet soda gained almost triple the abdominal fat over nine years as those who didn't. *Triple!* How is that possible? After all, doesn't diet soda have zero calories? Our developing understanding is that artificial sweeteners trigger sweetness receptors in the brain, which cause the body to prepare itself for an influx of calories. But when people drink diet soda, those calories never enter the body, so the body still craves them. Those cravings can cause you to ultimately eat more calories overall, putting you at risk for weight gain.

Instead of reaching for a diet soda, choose a naturally flavored (but unsweetened) club soda or carbonated water. There are so many options on the market now—in so many flavors—that there's really no reason to reach for that chemical-laden diet cola ever again.

Speaking of no-calorie seltzers, I'm often asked if they're okay to drink. The research says they won't do your gut wall any damage. However, if your belly feels bad after drinking these, it's because they can cause bloating and gas—which are miserable if only temporary.

We also used to worry that seltzer could leach calcium from your bones, but the Framingham study, which involved thousands of people, found that fizzy soft drinks are the bad news here because they're loaded with bone-destroying sugar and phosphates. It turns out other sparkling drinks are just fine for your bones—and that's good news.

If you're really missing cola (and its caffeine), the Dr. Zevia brand is a natural, caffeinated, zero-calorie, zero-sugar alternative. It may not be a health food, but compared to the colas in the red and blue cans, it's a big step in the right direction.

Let's Stop Saying "Goal Weight"

As someone who was on the clinic floor for over twenty years, I look at certain patient numbers to help establish a baseline and offer some perspective—things like weight, body mass index, and waist-to-hip ratio. They're all helpful—but not one of them offers a gospel truth when it comes to what you should or should not weigh or look like. A naturopathic physician never just looks at score cards; we look at people. And when it comes to people, the truth is no magic number exists.

Tell me if you relate to this scenario: You currently weigh X pounds. And you want to weigh Y pounds. Y can feel like a huge pile of laundry you don't have the energy to fold so you just leave it sitting on top of the dryer. For the next week, you take what you need from that pile of unfolded clothes in the laundry room. The clothes never get folded.

When you let yourself become so fixated on your goal weight, and the goal weight feels like too overwhelming a task, you never even get started. What if you changed your goal weight? The extreme all or nothing mentality is a sneaky little psychological sabotage.

Your ideal shouldn't be a number you always have to chase—like what you weighed as a sophomore in high school when you could fit into your favorite pair of Levi's—and it definitely shouldn't be a line you keep moving lower and lower still. BMI calculators and tape-measure recording can be helpful, but neither tells the whole story. That magic BMI number of twenty-five, for example, doesn't account for whether your weight comes from muscle or fat. It doesn't consider your age, your genetics, or the size at which you feel most comfortable. Using waist-to-hip ratio to assess healthy bodies is another popular measure. In general, a waist size greater than thirty-five inches for a woman or forty inches for a man can signal trouble, but these numbers don't factor in the data that many women are naturally apple shaped. This is all a research-backed way of telling you that to find your je ne sais quoi, you have to control the goal-weight narrative.

Use your height, weight, BMI, and waist circumference as a baseline. Then in addition, ask yourself these questions, and answer honestly:

Do you feel strong at your current weight? Can you physically do all the things you need and want to do—and do them with ease and without pain?

Do you feel energetic at your current weight? Are you peppy nearly all day and still going strong in the evening?

Do you feel healthy at your current weight? Are you free from weight-related problems like sleep apnea, metabolic syndrome, diabetes, heart disease, high blood pressure, bad choles-terol levels, or joint pain?

Do you feel happy at your current weight? Do you enjoy buy-ing and showing off new clothes? Are you comfortable and confi-dent being seen? You don't have to be at your goal weight to answer yes to this—take a moment to think about what you do like about yourself and your appearance before you answer.

If your answer to all four questions is yes, that's a big clue that you're at a weight that works well for you—whether you're a size two, a size eight, or a size fourteen.

If the answer to any of them is no, if you're gaining lots of belly fat, adding a clothing size every decade, or feeling old and tired and unhappy with your appearance, you can work to reach a weight where you answer yes to all of these questions.

In anything we're trying to accomplish, we should meet our-selves in the middle. Whatever you say your goal weight is right now, cut that in half to get yourself started. And with every couple pounds you lose, re-ask yourself these four questions.

You can take off those extra pounds with my breakthrough nutrition plan and get back to a weight that's ideal—not according to the height-weight charts, BMI calculators, and tape measures, but according to you.

Friendly Fiber Reminder

Author and pastor John Mark Comer published a book in 2019 called *The Ruthless Elimination of Hurry*. His thesis was that hurry is the enemy of spiritual life. It made a lot of readers question how fast they were moving through life. Near the end of the book, he gave twenty tips to slow down. His first tip was so simple, that it was, in my mind, border-line revolutionary. His tip was to drive the speed limit. It made me stop and think, *Wow, why don't I?* It was thought provoking in a way most great health advice is: so obvious that it's almost inarguable. That's how I feel about the simplicity of telling you to eat fiber. It's not revolutionary, but when you stop to think about it, *do you* eat enough? The average person does not.

When you're pursuing digestive health and weight loss, eating more fiber is *always* a good starting point. Why? Because it nourishes the good bacteria in your gut. Our digestive enzymes don't break down the fiber from vegetables and other sources, so it passes through the digestive track—essentially becoming a moveable feast for gut microbes. And happy, well-fed gut microbes behave. They do their jobs not just in digestion, but in immune function, neurological messaging, and keeping your gut wall strong.

Oh yeah, and in helping you regulate your weight.

How much is enough? Women should have at least 25 to 30 grams a day. This typically means incorporating fiber into every meal and snack. For example, mixing a cup of berries and a tablespoon of chia seeds into a breakfast smoothie equals 13 grams of fiber. Half an avocado added to your lunch equals 5 grams. Adding a cup of Brussels sprouts to dinner equals 5 grams. And an ounce of almonds as a snack equals 4 grams. And voilà: you've reached your goal. Fruits and vegetables are the greatest ways to get more fiber—and they're rolled up with generous doses of essential vitamins and micronutrients, too.

Worried about Fruit?

With the recent rise in low-carb diets like keto, fruit has become something people fear will make them fat. Let's set the record straight! Is fruit making you fat?! The answer is a qualified no. Let me explain: Fructose is a form of sugar found in fruit, and it can be stored as fat. Fructose has been linked to increased belly fat, slowed metabolism, and overall weight gain. Plus, fructose can spike insulin levels, and the body has a hard time burning fat while insulin levels are elevated. Certain fruits like grapes, mangoes, and cherries are higher in sugar. And so, if you are already overweight, regularly eating high-sugar fruit can impede your weight loss.

Now here's the flip side: Fruit is high in fiber and high in antioxidants—two things that are vital for good health! These two reasons alone are enough for me to insist that you do *not* need to fear fruit. You can eat from this food group every day, in moderation. Two servings is a healthy target. If you're worried about sugar content, choose lower-sugar options like berries, apples, and citrus.

Nuts and Seeds

Nuts and seeds are a healthy, delicious, nutrient-rich part of the breakthrough plan. I want you to enjoy them—a little every day. But portions matter when it comes to foods that are this calorie-dense, so you'll want to make a habit of measuring them into a small dish instead of eating straight from a box, can, or bag. When patients come to me frustrated because they're doing all the right things but not seeing results, overdoing the nuts and seeds is often the problem.

Water, Water, Water

If you hiked to the top of the highest mountain to speak with the wisest sage about how best to lose extra, unhealthy weight, she would likely look you deep in the eyes and speak this incantation: *Hydrate. Hydrate. Hydrate.*

And she would be right. Water is a natural appetite suppressant. It raises your metabolism. It flushes toxins and waste from your body. It helps keep your cells healthy and happy. It is cheap and plentiful and perfect. If you don't love it straight, try it with lemon, cucumber, or in the form of tea or . . . *bone broth.* All excellent options to help you hit that target of half your body weight in ounces every single day.

Thermogenic Bone Broth

Bone broth, lemon juice, watercress, and cayenne have a thermogenic effect that boosts your metabolism while keeping you satisfied. Enjoy as often as you like.

PREP TIME: 3 min.
COOK TIME: 3 min. and 10 min. wait time
YIELD: 1 serving

1 cup Chicken Bone Broth (page 272) or store-bought

1 to 2 teaspoons freshly squeezed lemon juice

1 handful of watercress, coarsely chopped

Pinch of Celtic sea or pink Himalayan salt

Pinch of freshly ground black pepper

Pinch of ground cayenne pepper

In a small saucepan, add the bone broth and lemon juice. Bring to a boil over high heat. Add the watercress, cover, turn off the heat, and steep for about 10 minutes. Season with the salt, pepper, and cayenne.

NOTE
To make the broth more filling, add 1 scoop collagen peptides.

Pot of Gold: Creamy Asparagus Soup

Asparagus offers many serious health perks. It helps promote overall digestive health due to its abundance of soluble and insoluble fiber. It's a natural diuretic and helps flush excess liquid from your body. Asparagus is also loaded with folic acid, vitamins, and minerals. It's easy to understand why it should be a staple in your weight-loss journey.

PREP TIME: 15 min.
COOK TIME: 25 min.
YIELD: 4 to 5 servings

2 tablespoons ghee or pasture-raised butter

2 leeks (white part only), thinly sliced

3 celery stalks, sliced

1 garlic clove, minced

1 quart (4 cups) Chicken Bone Broth (page 272) or store-bought

1 pound asparagus, cut into 1-inch pieces (tough ends discarded)

1 (14-ounce) can unsweetened full-fat coconut milk

Pinch of ground nutmeg, plus more for serving

1 teaspoon Celtic sea or pink Himalayan salt

$1/_2$ teaspoon freshly ground black pepper, plus more for serving

1 teaspoon arrowroot blended with 1 tablespoon water (see Notes)

In a large stockpot over medium heat, melt the ghee. Add the leeks and celery and sauté for 6 to 8 minutes to soften. Add garlic and sauté for another 1 to 2 minutes. Increase the heat to medium-high and add the bone broth and asparagus. When the soup begins to simmer, reduce the heat to medium and simmer for 15 to 20 minutes or until the asparagus is tender.

Purée the soup with an immersion blender, food processor, or blender until smooth (see Notes). Return the soup to the stockpot, stir in coconut milk, nutmeg, salt, pepper, and arrowroot. Simmer until soup has warmed through and thickens, adding more arrowroot if a thicker soup is desired. Serve warm with additional nutmeg and pepper to taste.

Key ingredients for weight loss: bone broth, garlic, celery, leeks, asparagus

NOTES

Arrowroot is a great gluten-free thickener, but it doesn't hold up well to reheating. Optionally, if you want to thicken when reheating, add about $1/_8$ to $1/_4$ teaspoon per serving and warm on the stovetop.

If you use a blender or food processor, process in batches, covering the top with a clean kitchen towel to avoid getting burned.

Pot of Gold: Broth with Mighty Greens

If you are trying to drop weight, this soup is my magic potion. Loaded with nutritious greens that are satisfying and very filling, you can enjoy this as a meal or between meals if you're feeling hungry. Keep a quart in the refrigerator so you always have it on hand—this helps keep life simple. Plus, you can make this recipe your own in countless ways. I've included a few variation suggestions in the notes to get you started.

PREP TIME: 15 min.
COOK TIME: 20 min.
YIELD: 6 to 8 servings

2 quarts (8 cups) Chicken Bone Broth (page 272) or store-bought

2 leeks (white parts only), thinly sliced

3 celery stalks, sliced

2 garlic cloves, minced or smashed

1 teaspoon dried tarragon or thyme, or 3 to 4 sprigs fresh

6 cups greens, plus more as desired, cut into $1/2$-inch ribbons (see Notes)

1 teaspoon Celtic sea or pink Himalayan salt

$1/2$ teaspoon freshly ground black pepper

Extra-virgin olive oil, for drizzling

In a large stockpot, combine the broth, leeks, celery, garlic, and tarragon. Simmer over medium heat for 8 to 10 minutes while the leeks soften and the herbs infuse the broth. Add the greens, salt, and pepper and simmer over low heat for 5 to 10 minutes until the greens are soft but not mushy. (If you are using collard greens, which take longer to cook, add them first and simmer until they begin to soften, then add the remaining greens.) Taste to adjust the seasonings and drizzle with the olive oil before serving.

Key ingredients for weight loss: bone broth, garlic, leeks, celery, greens

NOTES

You have a wide range of options for greens depending on your preferences—spinach, watercress, kale, cabbage, arugula, chard, collards, parsley, and cilantro are all great choices.

Depending on the greens you select, make sure to remove the tough stems and center veins before chopping into ribbons.

If you prefer your soup smooth and creamy, purée with an immersion blender, food processor, or blender. If you use a blender or food processor, process in batches, covering the top with a clean kitchen towel to avoid getting burned. Optionally, you can add full-fat coconut milk (from a can) to make this soup creamier.

Feel free to add any of your favorite herbs or spices. I like mine with freshly ground black pepper, a pinch of cayenne pepper, and a dash of hot sauce.

For extra protein in your soup, add cooked chicken, chicken or turkey sausage, or meatballs (about 4 to 5 ounces per serving).

Add a squeeze of fresh lemon or lime juice. Lime juice is especially pleasing if you use cilantro.

Try topping with diced avocado before you drizzle with the olive oil.

Pot of Gold: Spicy Seafood Soup (Caldo de Mariscos)

This is quite possibly my favorite soup of all time. It's so good that I created the recipe with 8 to 10 servings because it gets better and better as it sits. Plus, if you made half as much, you'd just need to make it again! It's based on a traditional Mexican recipe called "caldo de mariscos." It has a depth of flavor that is hard to

PREP TIME: 20 min.
COOK TIME: 25 min.
YIELD: 8 to 10 servings

describe because of the complex blend of herbs, spices, and chiles. The ingredient list is long, but don't be discouraged. Each of the components adds to the robust flavor. It's not difficult to make; it will just take a few more minutes to measure the seasonings than some of the other recipes in this book. But rest assured, your time will be well spent. And this one is bursting with metabolism-boosting ingredients!

2 dried guajillo chiles, cut in half vertically (stems and seeds removed; see Notes)

1$^1/_2$ tablespoons extra-virgin olive oil

1 medium onion cut into $^1/_2$-inch dice or 2 leeks (white parts only), thinly sliced

2 celery stalks, cut into $^1/_2$-inch dice

3 carrots, cut into $^1/_2$-inch dice

3 large garlic cloves, minced

2 teaspoons ground cumin

1$^1/_2$ teaspoons ancho chile powder

$^1/_2$ teaspoon dried thyme

$^1/_2$ teaspoon dried oregano

$^1/_2$ teaspoon dried marjoram

1 tablespoon Celtic sea or pink Himalayan salt

$^1/_2$ teaspoon freshly ground black pepper

1$^1/_2$ quarts (6 cups) Chicken Bone Broth (page 272) or store-bought

1 (28-ounce) can fire-roasted tomatoes

5 pounds cod or other firm white fish, cut into 2-inch chunks

2 tablespoons fresh cilantro, plus more for serving (stems removed)

Lime wedges, for serving, optional

Sliced avocado, for serving, optional

In a small saucepan over low heat, add the guajillo chiles and 1 cup of water and simmer for about 8 minutes to soften. If the water level gets low, add enough water so the chiles stay immersed.

In a large stockpot over medium heat, add the olive oil, onions, celery, and carrots and sauté for about 5 minutes. Add the garlic, cumin, chile powder, thyme, oregano, marjoram, salt, and pepper and stir to combine. Add the bone broth, cover, and simmer for about 8 minutes.

In a blender or food processor, add the tomatoes and the softened chiles (along with any remaining water) and purée until smooth. Add the tomato mixture to the stockpot. Stir to combine and bring to a simmer over medium-low heat. Add the cod and simmer for 5 to 7 minutes or until the fish flakes.

Add the cilantro, stir, and taste to adjust the seasonings. Serve with more cilantro, the lime wedges, and the avocado slices (if using, which is traditional).

Key ingredients to support weight loss: bone broth, garlic, chiles, chile powder

---

NOTES

Guajillo chiles have a sweet, fruity, and somewhat smoky flavor, and when fresh, they are called the Mirasol chile. Guajillo chiles have a mild heat, registering 2,500 to 5,000 on the Scoville scale and are commonly used in Mexican cooking. You can buy dried whole guajillo chiles, usually pre-bagged, in Mexican grocery stores.

For added spice, add more ancho chile powder or 1 to 2 pinches of ground cayenne pepper.

You can also use any other seafood or a combination of seafood, such as shrimp, clams, mussels, scallops, calamari, or octopus. If you use shellfish, be sure to scrub the shells.

Eat within 2 days. You can freeze for up to 4 months in a tightly sealed container.

Pot of Gold: Italian Vegetable Soup with Sausage and Fennel

Italian vegetable soup is such a homey, comforting classic. There are as many recipes for vegetable soup as there are cooks, so feel free to add any of your favorite non-starchy vegetables or remove any you don't favor. I'm particularly fond of fennel because it has such a lovely mild anise flavor that mellows and softens as it cooks, adding a rich depth of flavor and a subtle sweetness to the soup.

PREP TIME: 15 min.
COOK TIME: 45 min.
YIELD: 8 servings

2 tablespoons extra-virgin olive oil, divided, plus more for drizzling

1 pound nitrate- and sugar-free natural Italian turkey or chicken sausage, sliced into $1/_2$-inch-thick pieces

2 leeks (white part only), thinly sliced

1 fennel bulb, thinly sliced

4 garlic cloves, minced

2 quarts (8 cups) Chicken Bone Broth (page 272) or store-bought

2 dried bay leaves

3 carrots, cut into circles

2 celery stalks, thinly sliced

$1/_4$ cup loosely packed fresh basil leaves (stems removed)

3 cups packed baby spinach or Swiss chard

1 to 2 teaspoons Celtic sea or pink Himalayan salt

$1/_2$ teaspoon freshly ground black pepper

Crushed red pepper flakes, for serving, optional

In a stockpot over medium heat, add 1 tablespoon of the olive oil and the sausage and sauté until it is no longer pink inside, 10 to 12 minutes. Remove the sausage from the pot, add the remaining 1 tablespoon olive oil, the leeks, and fennel and sauté for about 10 minutes. Add the garlic and sauté for 1 minute. Add the broth, bay leaves, carrots, and celery, increase the heat to medium-high, and bring to a simmer. Reduce heat to medium-low and simmer for 15 to 20 minutes or until the carrots are tender. Add the basil and spinach and continue to simmer for another 3 to 5 minutes to wilt the greens. Season with the salt and pepper and remove the bay leaves. Drizzle with the olive oil and garnish with the pepper flakes (if using).

Key ingredients to support weight loss: bone broth, lean meat, leeks, fennel, garlic, celery, basil, spinach and/or chard, red pepper flakes

Berry Chia Parfait

Chia seeds have been touted for their health benefits for centuries. They were an important food source for both the Maya and Aztec cultures of Mexico and Central America. Two tablespoons of chia seeds have almost 10 grams of fiber. That's around 40% of the recommended daily intake. Because of that they are very satiating and will keep you feeling full for a long time.

PREP TIME: 10 min. and 30-plus min. wait time

YIELD: 4 servings

They are also highly nutritious and contain antioxidants, protein, B vitamins, omega-3s, and linoleic acid. This parfait is incredibly satisfying for breakfast or dessert.

1 quart (4 cups) almond, coconut, cashew, or other unsweetened nut milk

1 teaspoon vanilla extract

Stevia or monk fruit sweetener equal to 3 tablespoons sugar (see Notes)

8 to 12 tablespoons chia seeds (see Notes)

$1/4$ to $1/2$ teaspoon ground cinnamon, optional

2 cups blueberries, raspberries, blackberries, sliced strawberries, or any combination

In a mixing bowl, combine the milk, vanilla, sweetener, chia seeds, and cinnamon (if using). Mix well and refrigerate for at least 30 minutes. It's even better if you can chill it overnight.

To assemble the parfaits, spoon $1/2$ cup of the chia pudding into each of four 14-ounce canning jars or glasses, top each with $1/4$ cup of the berries, another $1/2$ cup of the chia pudding, and the remaining berries. Cover and refrigerate.

Key ingredients to support weight loss: chia, berries

NOTES

Know your sweetener: Depending on what form of sweetener you purchase, you'll need to find the conversion (either on the package or online) that equals the amount called for in the recipe.

If you've never made chia pudding, you'll quickly see that chia seeds, when mixed in a liquid, turn into a texture resembling pudding. Sometimes the seeds will form clumps, so mix well when you combine them with the nut milk, and again after being refrigerated. Two tablespoons in a cup of milk will create a pudding-like texture, but if you like a thicker pudding, you can add additional seeds.

If you don't want to go through the trouble of layering parfaits, just put fruit on the top of the pudding and enjoy!

Halibut with Romesco Sauce

Originating in Catalonia, Spain, history has it that fishermen created romesco sauce for their catch. And like many sauces from around the world, while romesco has some basic ingredients, every cook makes it specific to her own liking. This incredibly simple sauce might appear to have a long list of ingredients, but you probably have most of them in your pantry. Just put everything in a food processor and press start.

PREP TIME: 15 min.

COOK TIME (FOR THE FISH): 12 min.

YIELD: 2$^1/_2$ to 3 cups sauce, enough for 4-plus halibut fillets

1 (8- to 10-ounce) jar roasted red peppers, drained

1 (14-ounce) can diced fire-roasted tomatoes, drained

$^1/_4$ cup extra-virgin olive oil

1 cup toasted almonds, hazelnuts, pine nuts, or a combination

2 to 3 garlic cloves, minced

2 tablespoons freshly squeezed lemon juice

1 teaspoon sherry or red wine vinegar

1 teaspoon ground smoked paprika

$^1/_2$ teaspoon crushed red pepper flakes, plus more as needed

$^1/_2$ teaspoon Celtic sea or pink Himalayan salt, plus more as needed

$^1/_4$ teaspoon freshly ground black pepper

$^1/_4$ cup fresh Italian parsley (stems removed), optional

1 (4- to 6-ounce) halibut fillet per person

Avocado oil, for brushing

Place an oven rack in the center of the oven and preheat it to 425°F. Line a baking dish or sheet pan with parchment paper for easy clean up (optional), and set aside.

To make the romesco, in a food processor, combine the red peppers, tomatoes, olive oil, almonds, garlic, lemon juice, vinegar, paprika, red pepper flakes, salt, pepper, and parsley (if using) and blend until the mixture is smooth but still has some texture. Taste to adjust the seasonings as desired.

To make the halibut, rinse the fillets in cold water and dry with paper towels. Place the halibut fillets in the baking dish. Brush or spray the fillets with the avocado oil. Bake for 10 to 12 minutes or until the fish is opaque and flakes with a fork. The fillets should reach an internal temperature of 145°F.

To serve, generously top the halibut with 2 or more tablespoons of the romesco sauce.

Key ingredients to support weight loss: fish, crushed red pepper flakes, nuts, garlic, lemon

---

NOTES

You can also use cod or any other firm-flesh white fish.

You will have some sauce left over if you don't also top everything else on your plate with it (which is tempting). Enjoy it with chicken, lamb, vegetables, and just about anything else.

Lemon Chicken, Asparagus, and Leeks with Pan Sauce

This is a quick and easy dinner you can whip up in about 35 minutes. Leeks and asparagus are a match made in food heaven, and lemon adds a refreshing burst of citrus. Yum! Plus the sauce is outrageously delicious because you make it by deglazing the pan. And since you make the entire dinner in one pan, cleanup is easy, too.

PREP TIME: 15 min.
COOK TIME: 20 min.
YIELD: 4 servings

This is a dish that tastes decadent, but it is packed with quality protein, fibrous veggies, alliums, and, of course, bone broth—a yes even when you're working hard to lose weight.

1 pound boneless, skinless chicken breasts (see Notes)

1 teaspoon Celtic sea or pink Himalayan salt

$1/_2$ teaspoon freshly ground black pepper

3 tablespoons ghee or pasture-raised butter, divided (see Notes)

3 leeks (white parts only), sliced into $1/_2$-inch circles

1 to 2 garlic cloves, minced

1 pound asparagus, cut into 1-inch pieces (tough ends discarded)

$1/_2$ cup Chicken Bone Broth (page 272) or store-bought

1 tablespoon freshly squeezed lemon juice

$1/_4$ cup Italian flat leaf parsley, coarsely chopped

Cut the chicken breasts into cutlets (see Notes) and season with the salt and pepper.

In a large sauté pan over medium-high heat, melt 1 tablespoon of the ghee. When the pan is hot, sauté several cutlets for 3 to 4 minutes on each side, just until just cooked through and golden. Be mindful not to overcrowd the pan. The internal temperature should reach 165°F. Remove the first batch of cutlets from pan, add another 1 tablespoon of the ghee and cook the remaining chicken in batches. Cover the chicken and set aside.

In the same pan over medium heat, add the remaining 1 tablespoon ghee and sauté the leeks for about 5 minutes. Add the garlic and asparagus and sauté for another 5 minutes. Spread the mixture over the chicken, cover, and set aside.

Add the bone broth and lemon juice to the pan and deglaze (see Notes). Stir in the parsley and spoon the pan sauce over the chicken and asparagus.

Key ingredients supporting weight loss: bone broth, lean meat (chicken breast), garlic, leeks, asparagus, lemon, parsley

NOTES

If chicken cutlets are not available at the grocery store, you can slice them at home using this technique, which works well for chicken breasts that are oversized (8 to 10 ounces each). By slicing them horizontally into cutlets, you end up with two thinner breast fillets. To do so, be sure the chicken is very cold or just thawed. You can put them in the freezer on a plate (not stacked) for 10 to 15 minutes if needed. Place a cold chicken breast on a cutting board with the smooth side up. Hold it in place with the palm of your hand, keeping your hand flat on top of the breast. Using a sharp knife, start at the thickest end and slice the breast in half horizontally, cutting toward the thinner end. You should have two chicken breast cutlets that are 4 to 5 ounces each. You don't need to slice smaller (4- to 5-ounce) chicken breasts. Optionally, if you want the cutlets even thinner, place them between two sheets of waxed paper or plastic wrap and pound with a meat mallet to the desired thickness.

It's best to use ghee if you have it on hand because the milk solids have been removed (it's essentially clarified butter), and it won't burn like butter. You can also use avocado oil, but the flavor of the ghee or butter is what makes the pan sauce so luscious.

To deglaze the pan, place it over medium to medium-high heat, add the liquid, and bring to a boil. Use a wooden spoon to scrape up the browned bits in the pan. Reduce the heat to medium-low and simmer for 5 to 8 minutes until the liquid is reduced by half.

Chapter 9

Fired Up: From Sick and Tired to Healthy and Energized

E ven if feeling sick and tired isn't a regular part of your life (and I hope it's not), we all go through phases when we get run down and our health begins to feel fragile. For me, as for many moms, the ultimate example of this occurred when my kids were little. When I delivered my first son, labor was long and hard. Two years later, my second son came rushing into the world in four hours flat. Even though they are eighteen and twenty now, both headed to the Coast Guard (humble mom brag right there!), I remember those years when I was a young mother like they were yesterday. I was flooded with overwhelming love for my babies. I *constantly* worried about them. I had a postpartum body I didn't recognize. I endured sleepless night after sleepless night. And all the while, I was struggling to keep my career and marriage afloat.

I distinctly remember a morning when I was running late, and as I ran out the door with my hair on fire, one of my boys stretched his arms toward me, saying, "Mom, Mom." Of course, he didn't want me to go. And, of course, I had to do it. I couldn't stay one second longer because my patients would be waiting.

Morning after morning in those early years, I hurried away in chaos. Like nearly every mom I know, I did what I had to do—even when it was more than *anyone* could realistically balance. It's no surprise I hit a wall. I look at photos of me from that time, and all I can think is how low I *felt*, how low I *looked*. My eyes were sunken, my skin pale, my waist expanded, my hair clipped with extensions to mask how thin it was getting. The pressure and exhaustion I felt were constantly weighing me down.

Technically, mathematically, I was supposed to be in a sweet spot, prime moment, in a woman's life. High energy. Making high-powered moves in the workplace. High sex drive. High on life. But the truth? I was at the bottom. I caught every little cough and cold that crossed my path. I looked old and felt tired. I didn't even want to *think* about sex. My tank was empty.

What I wanted, what I craved day after day, was some way, *any* way, of feeling restored and energized again. I had gone into all of it—motherhood, career, relationships, homes, friendships—fired up and so excited, but in those first years of trying to keep it all going, I burned out.

In my decades of clinical practice, there was one gut-punch statement I heard from new patients far too often—one that always snapped me back to those challenging days and compelled me to make helping them my highest calling. That statement was, *I feel dead inside.* It set off alarm bells in my system every time. I knew that when a patient felt this way, they were in trouble. Sometimes this was indicative of depression. But often, these patients had reached an ultimate place of exhaustion—a point where they were going through the motions of their lives, feeling like cardboard cutouts of themselves.

Many of these women (and sometimes men) were already sick by the time I met them. Others were at a tipping point where they'd ceased to take their physical and emotional needs seriously. The effects were starting to show. And a few were still pushing back on fatigue—forcing themselves to meet obligations that felt like too much, trying to borrow on reserves of energy that were long empty. In cases like this, fatigue is sometimes the problem, but often it's a symptom of something bigger. Either way, when it starts plaguing your life, it's time to put on your detective cap and investigate where things went wrong so you can get back on the road to good health and positive energy.

If you're wondering where the line is—how to decide whether you're just tired or whether you're dealing with more serious fatigue—a good night's sleep or a relaxing weekend should give you the answer. When you're worn down in a plain-old-tired way, sleep is a fix. When you're bone-tired every day for weeks or months on end, something bigger is going on. And when your exhaustion impacts you, both physically and mentally, for long periods, it may be time to consult with your doctor for a deeper investigation. If you don't have a practitioner you love, I always recommend people to a functional medicine doctor, because they dig deep and get to root causes.

There are two main areas where I want you to look for both problems and solutions: the boundaries in your life and your gut health (yes, gut health is *directly* tied to your energy and immune health). We'll look at each, and then I'll share some energizing, immune-boosting foods and delicious recipes that can help nourish you and lift you up. Oh yes, and we'll talk about sex—because energy level and libido are deeply connected, and I want you to have plenty of both.

But first, we need to talk about how all these threads tie together— why the unraveling of one almost always ends up impacting the others.

The Energy-Immunity-Gut (and Bone Broth!) Connection

I often advise patients to look at their bodies like they would a New York City subway map—because everything has a way of connecting underground. Your body's systems are intimately intertwined, and nowhere is this more true than in the relationships between your energy level, your immune system, and your gut health.

Consider the facts:

- That gut microbiome we talked about in chapter 7 and your immune system are in constant contact and mutual support to help you stay healthy. The good bacteria in your gut help your immune cells learn to identify when your body is threatened with disease or infection—and they also help your immune system adapt to long-term changes. Studies estimate that as much as 70% (or more!) of your immune function is based in the gut.
- Exhaustion and the stress it causes (much more about stress in chapter 10) can decrease the number of lymphocytes in your body. These are the cells your immune system deploys when it encounters viral disease. Think of them as your antiviral army—an army you need to stay combat ready. Ever get a cold sore when you're stressed? Or come home sick after an overwhelming work trip? That's likely because a drop in your lymphocyte levels put you at higher risk for viruses, including the common cold and cold sores.
- One upshot of these relationships is that your body *needs* sleep to fight infectious diseases. Long-term lack of sleep also increases your risk of obesity, diabetes, and heart and blood vessel (cardiovascular) disease.
- Paradoxically, if you're always tired, it is sometimes a consequence of your immune system working *too hard*—flooding the body with messengers that can play a role in the many conditions we call autoimmune diseases.
- It can be difficult for some kinds of immune cells to regain their strength and effectiveness once they become exhausted. Like microcosms of our whole bodies, once they're worn down, they get used to a new normal.
- Wondering what all of this has to do with *bone broth*? Here are three reasons to keep it on the menu every day:

1. Making bone broth a regular part of your diet is one of the biggest keys to boosting gut health—which in turn empowers your immune system to do good work.

2. Our bodies have specialized immune cells called "T cells," which convert sugar into energy. Glutamine, one of the main proteins that make up the collagen in bone broth, is required for these cells to function.

3. Bone broth gives you a rich dose of "conditional amino acids"—glycine, proline, arginine, and (again!) glutamine—that your adrenal glands need to heal themselves if they're burned out. These are amino acids that your body can't supply in adequate quantities if it's run-down.

Boundaries and the Lemon Tree Problem

A friend of mine moved into a new home with a magnificent lemon tree—a tree that takes decades to grow—in the backyard. It was beautiful, but it produced only one lemon every couple weeks. As my friend drove around her new Southern California town and past other lemon trees that were bursting with fruit, she wondered why hers was the Charlie Brown tree? She suspected that it was dying, and in a last-ditch effort to save it, she called a botanist. The botanist took one look at the tree and reported that its roots were being suffocated by its landscaping. In less than an hour, he'd pushed back the layer of rocks around the trunk and removed layers of heavy weed barrier as well. After finishing, he said the tree would be able to "breathe." Then he added fertilizer and new mulch so it could grow.

Within a year, the "dying" lemon tree was bursting with blossoms and then with fruit.

I loved hearing this story because it felt like an allegory describing my life's work as a naturopathic physician. When a patient is failing to thrive, I look for clues as to what's going on. I help guide them to clear away the life layers that are suffocating them and undermining their health. And together, we construct new regimens to overcome obstacles to health. In the naturopathic framework, focusing solely on the end symptoms is never enough. True healing comes when you also address the terrain in which disease developed.

Now make no mistake, the conditions in which that lemon tree was struggling to thrive were *going to* lead to disease. It was stifled; it was working endlessly but hardly bearing fruit; it was—for a tree—*exhausted* in every sense of the word. But the moment it was given some much-needed TLC, it was on the brink of going another way—of beginning a trajectory away from illness.

But we aren't really talking about lemon trees anymore, are we? We're talking about you, and about why you sometimes get so tired that it's a struggle to put your feet on the floor at the start of a new day and set out into the world again.

In chapter 6, we talked about stamina-care, a favorite topic for me. But in the context of an energy crisis—your energy crisis—it's important to home in on what this means and what you can do to ease the fatigue factors in your life. The fact is women have been putting others' needs before their own for centuries—probably forever. For starters, it's the nature of motherhood, because those babies aren't gonna take care of themselves. But what about before, or after as our children become able to do things for themselves? I know women ranging in age from eighteen to ninety-eight who shunt off their own needs for those of the people around them, sacrificing rest, fun, friends, or sex. When you tally it up, we are talking about lifetimes of sacrifice—just entirely too much.

The pandemic cemented this truth for anyone who was in doubt. Women were forced to do it all and the world took note. Work from home, parent while working, teach while parenting—all while making tough decisions about the states of their finances and the safety of their families. As if by default, it fell largely to women to modify everything about our lives, to integrate work and caregiving—to make it work. And although we were already doing this, the pandemic elevated our pressures to a new level—and exposed to everyone that women truly put their needs after everyone else's.

We got through it—of course. We are strong. But many of the women in my life are still shell-shocked by the demands of life before, during, and after the pandemic. And each of us owes it to ourselves to stop periodically—at least once a month—to self-assess how we're doing. To ask if the day's exhaustion is because it's well past bedtime or because we're rapidly approaching a burnout.

Feeling fatigued is the ultimate symptom of self-neglect. Deciding to turn the switch back on for your body, to figure out what it's going to take to flood light and life back into your matrix of energy, is the only solution.

Sometimes we just need to get moving—to remember that exercise is the great cure-all for so many problems in our lives. But burnout fatigue is a different kind of crisis. You feel it deeply. You may notice other signs of fatigue—thinning hair, dark circles, increased anxiety, quick temper, low energy at night. In the past, maybe you didn't mind going out once in a while, but now it's such a heavy lift that you can't be bothered. If you're in a relationship, maybe you used to seek out intimacy with your partner but now just seek your pillow. If you're actively single, maybe you used to seek out a partner but now just seek your pillow.

Think you're just being a weenie? I doubt it. But test it out. Push a little more on a single aspect of your life, like going for a walk or out to dinner with a friend. When you do it, does it energize you? Or does it leave you feeling even emptier?

Identify the Culprits

This brings us to an important self-assessment that I call the *Five Ws of Fatigue*. I want you to consider them as if the stakes are high. Be honest with yourself so you can start figuring out ways to get your energy level back up where it belongs.

1. Who is stealing most of your mental energy? Is it a child who's on the wrong track? A boss who you've been trying to please for years? A spouse you have to walk on eggshells around? A friendship? A deep moral dilemma? A secret?

2. What is causing you to physically feel fatigued? A demanding job that you're working sixty hours a week at just to keep up? A household where nobody but you pitches in to get everything done? A chaotic schedule where you're constantly running from one place to the next? A poor diet? Extra weight?

3. When does fatigue hit you the hardest? In the morning when you're hitting snooze because you cannot get out of bed? At night when you crash under the pressure of the next day? On the weekends, which feel like a whirlwind of obligations? The minute you sit at your desk to start working? The minute your kids walk in the door after school?

4. Where in your life do you feel the most drained? Where does fatigue play out in your life? What parts of your life suffer the most from your fatigue? Home? Work? Your relationships?

5. Why has your fatigue been getting worse? Are you scared of failure? Are you scared to speak up? Are you in financial trouble? Are you scared to be alone? Are you frustrated by an inability to stick to a nutrition or fitness program?

Knowing what is draining you is the first step in finding a more energetic path. Answering these questions gives you the authority to start dealing with these burdens, one by one. What can you let go of? What can you solve? What can you make peace with in your life? What do you acknowledge is a trade for something you believe is worth any sacrifice? You don't have to clear cut the forest of your worries and trials, but today is a good day to start pruning concerns, one by one, until they begin to feel more manageable.

Making Changes

Life demands a lot from you. No one is immune to the pressure. No matter if you're a rock star performing in shows every other day, a triage nurse working twelve-hour shifts, or a mom spending hours in a pickup and drop-off line, you're often pushing your limits.

The remedy for this is always going to come down to sleep, nutrition, and stamina-care—so it's imperative that you make room for them in your life. You know I'm all about transformations—they are the foundation of my career and the work of which I'm most proud. Well, I need to tell you that sometimes transformation is as much about what you give up as it is about what you adopt. When you are sick and tired and need to find a way to get fired up again, I want you to create a new kind of list—the reverse to-do list. I call it a no-need-to-do list.

It hinges on one simple question: what can you take *off* your plate today that will make room for something that supports your health, energy, spirit, and/or immune system?

A few examples:

- Do you have to go to your cousin's daughter's second wedding's bridal shower? Bailing on this obligatory event could free up time for you to take a yoga class you've been wanting to try.
- Do you have to go to happy hour for an acquaintance's birthday? Skipping that could give you an opportunity to take a long soaking bath after work.
- Do you have to show up for that pointless meeting about how to use the new projector in the conference room? Taking a personal day you've earned could free up time for you to sleep in or take a nap.
- Do you have to shop for a new dress for an upcoming wedding or hit three different stores to clear your grocery list? Letting go of unnecessary errands can free up time to read or meditate.
- Do you and your spouse need an elaborate home-cooked meal or is it okay to make eggs for dinner and call it a night? Taking the simpler route could give you both the opportunity to take a leisurely after-dinner walk.

If you don't already have a no-need-to-do list, I suggest starting one now.

Pains of Change

I wish I could tell you that addressing those energy drains in your life is easy, that you'll always find sunshine and flowers immediately on the other side of hard choices. But we all know that's not the truth. Change—even change for the better—can come with pains of adjustment, pains of acceptance, and pain over the things we give up.

In this book, one of the themes I've come back to repeatedly is one I believe from the bottom of my heart: As you decide what you will eat, whether you will work out, when you will sleep, whether you are worthy of setting aside time for a long walk or a hot bath or a day to just relax and reset—I wish for you to always come from the mindset of *choosing*, not *cheating*. You want the slice of chocolate cake, you have the freedom to *choose* that. You want a nap instead of a workout today: another choice. You're just fine being a mom who buys goods for the school bake sale instead of spending her Saturday in the kitchen? Another choice. And some of the hardest choices we all have to make come down to boundaries.

When the choices you have to make are about people, about personal commitments, that's when it can really get hard. I am going to get more vulnerable than usual here and make a confession: I often suffer from loneliness. When I'm honest with myself, I admit that it sometimes makes my heart ache. Why, when I have a business and family and friends, do I feel this way? Because throughout my life, as I've prioritized my patients, my business, and my brand, and followed what I believe is my calling to be a leader in the world of wellness, there have been relationships I've sacrificed or given less to than I might have if I'd chosen a different path. I *chose* to follow a calling. And I've accepted that sometimes that pursuit brings loneliness.

When it kicks in, I've learned I have two options. I can succumb to it, wallow in a pity party for one, maybe even go to a dark place or reach for vices that don't serve me, like food or alcohol. *Or* I can choose to do something productive, to ground myself in my *why* and in the precious relationships that do meet my high bar for priority.

Setting boundaries is often the hardest part of transformation. But doing so is *how* you water your roots to give yourself life.

Are You Inflamm-aging?

In the simplest sense of the word, *inflammation* is a good thing. When your body feels threatened by invaders like bacteria, toxins, or an injury, your immune cells activate inflammatory cells to protect you from these attackers. Think of your immune cells like a 911 dispatcher who sends first responders (those ever-reliable inflammatory cells) to the scene. We love our inflammatory cells. They can quite literally be lifesavers. They can trap bacteria or begin work to heal injuries.

But when a threat passes and they're no longer needed for your *immediate* protection—they need to stand down.

Rush-to-the-scene-and-save-the-day inflammation is not a problem. What *is* a problem is chronic inflammation. It's what happens when inflammatory cells are activated by your body when you're *not* sick or injured—when they show up, make camp, and keep your systems on high alert. Think of a burglar alarm: A windowpane breaks, the alarm goes off, the thief runs away, the police do a report—and you go back to bed. But have you ever had to live—even for a matter of hours—with a malfunctioning alarm? One that goes off repeatedly for no good reason or can't be shut down?

At that point, it's not a tool for you to use—it's a source of trouble, stress, anxiety, and exhaustion.

Lifestyle factors, including chronic stress, being overweight, smoking, excessive drinking, environmental toxins, and a poor diet high in fried, processed, and over-sweetened foods all contribute to this chronic inflammation. They tamper with your body's alarm system, and, in the process, they wear you down.

This is why you often hear nutrition professionals advise you to eat a diet that is anti-inflammatory. And yes, the nutrition plan I laid out in chapter 3 is a powerful tool in reversing chronic inflammation.

In 2000, Italian immunology professor Claudio Franceschi introduced the theory of "inflamm-aging," a term which links inflammation with major age-related diseases, such as Alzheimer's disease, atherosclerosis, heart disease, type 2 diabetes, and cancer.

What does it mean for you? Be kind and nurturing to your immune system and your gut, and you can actually reverse inflammation and help prevent the age-related diseases you fear most.

Speaking of Getting Fired Up . . . Let's Talk about Libido

I would be remiss if I dug into the topic of energy without touching on what it means for sex. There is a stereotype that runs rampant in our society: that men *always* want sex and that women *never* do. Perhaps that's why so many women who confide in me about their lack of sex drive feel ashamed about it.

It's time to change this narrative because it just isn't true. Women go through phases where we crave sex, and we go through phases where we'd rather eat dirt. Most of us go through both at one time or another. The fact is *women's bodies are designed to constantly change.* We gain—and then lose—forty-plus pounds (often multiple times) to have children. We endure weight fluctuations monthly when menstruating. The size of our breasts fluctuates throughout our lives. And after the first fifty years or so, Mother Nature says, *Oh no, I'm not done,* and pushes us into menopause with a whole new world of changes.

What a woman's body is capable of is beautiful and amazing with a capital *A*, and the ever-changing nature of our shapes undoubtedly contributes to our ever-changing libido. This is why I hate the stereotype that men always want sex and women never do. How ridiculous. In hearing from thousands of patients over decades, what I've come to realize is that, just like almost everything else in our lives, *sex has seasons.* Women ebb in and out of wanting sex, needing it, hating it, or, frankly, being repulsed by it.

And let's be honest, ladies, a lot of the time when we're "not in the mood," our reasons come down to the same thing we've been talking about throughout this chapter: we are *exhausted.* I challenge you to find an adult woman who has not, at some point in her life, simply been too fatigued to have or enjoy sex. She may be out there, like a unicorn, but I haven't met her yet.

This is why, when a woman comes to me and opens up about a loss of interest in sex, I'm able to tell her with confidence that a lack of sex drive isn't the problem; it's a symptom of something else going on in her life or in her body. Sometimes the root cause is obvious—like an impossibly demanding schedule, a strained relationship, or a physical illness. Often it's a combination of factors.

Why are we talking about this in a book about wellness breakthroughs? Simple: the role of a naturopathic physician is to help guide patients toward overall, natural health. Rest assured there are few aspects of the human condition more relevant than sexual health. The fact is, there are so many reasons why sex can be the ultimate wellness booster that it's worth it to count them:

1. Sex gets your heart pumping, circulating oxygen throughout your body.
2. Like other forms of exercise, sex lowers your blood pressure.

3. Sex is a natural pain reliever.

4. Sex can boost immunity by raising antibody levels.

5. Sex makes you happy by flooding your body with feel-good hormones like oxytocin.

6. Sex helps you sleep better.

7. Sex begets more sex. Yep, when we block sex from our lives for extended periods of time, our hormone levels can wane. But this does not have to be permanent. Remember, there's a season for everything.

That's a pretty good start, don't you think?

Now let's talk about those common obstacles to a healthy sex life and what you can do to start finding that fire again:

1. Fatigue and stress. They're the two great slayers of desire. If you suffer from a lack of sleep or a pressure-filled schedule, neither your body nor your brain are working at top form—and neither is likely to have energy or interest for sex. Sex is, for many of us, what naturally follows when everything else is right with the world, when we feel good inside and out. That relaxed, happy sensibility can be nearly impossible to come by when you're exhausted or overburdened by anxiety. When you address your energy level in other areas of your life, your sexual energy is likely to follow.

2. Lack of body confidence. It can happen in any season of life, including pregnancy, exhaustion, a bout of stress eating, menopause, grief, illness, shifts in relationships, or any other change. It can reflect the way you actually appear or the way you are feeling about yourself. Regardless of the roots of these feelings, if you look in the mirror and can't feel love for the woman you see, that's a world-class libido buster. You can start addressing this on a daily basis with three steps: affirmations, exercise, and stamina-care. Choose one or choose them all, but I want you to do a little (or a lot) more for yourself. Push someone or something else to the back of the line. You deserve to feel good about the woman in the mirror. She is beautiful and full of light.

3. Tired relationships. Sometimes relationships become stale, sometimes they cycle back around to being fulfilling, and sometimes they come to an end. Too often, I meet women who are in relationship ruts. Maybe they're taken for granted or treated poorly; maybe they don't feel good about themselves and that impacts how they feel about their partners. Maybe they are looking for new partners and frustrated with how difficult it can be to find someone with whom they share a meaningful bond. In every case, there are women who beat themselves up for not wanting sex. Relationships have cycles, just like everything else in our lives, and when you're at a low point in one for any reason, it can feel like sex is just plain over and done.

If you've decided you don't *want* sex, or if you believe you have a perfectly healthy relationship in which it just happens once a year, don't feel badly for even a heartbeat about owning that decision. There is no more personal preference than whether you want to engage in any kind of intimacy. But if you are giving up on sex because that feels like your only option, or if you're just not sure . . . I have a litmus test to find out if you're really satisfied. I call it *50 Shades of DKA*, and it's simple. Read the book *50 Shades of Grey* or settle into an evening of *Bridgerton* or some equally racy television series. If you feel aroused while immersed in either, you have your answer. There is a reason why women across the world gobble up these tales of love and lust—because the need to be aroused is still deep within, alive and well.

That reason, friends, comes back to what inspires you. Women's libido is a complex topic, one that researchers have spent a lot of time investigating but rarely come to a consensus on, except for these consistent observations: It's complicated. It takes time. It is tied to intimacy as well as physicality. Like the stories of *50 Shades* and *Bridgerton*, it's fair to say many women prefer their sex lives to have a bit of a plot.

4. Shifting hormones. It's no secret that hormone levels shift as we age, including those of estrogen, progesterone, and testosterone—all of which can play a role in sexual arousal. But hear this: just because your hormone levels wane does not mean you've reached the end of your "hot" years, as long as you'd like them to continue. In fact, the idea that women lose interest in sex once they're past child-bearing age has been widely debunked. If you doubt, go ask a few friends with newly empty nests how their sex lives are going, and I guarantee some of those answers will curl your hair. Those years when women are theoretically supposed to be hanging up their sexuality? Studies tell us many women enjoy some of the best sex of their lives once the kids are grown and out of the house.

If you're wondering how that can be when hormone levels drop, the answer brings us back to seasons. Maybe your forties, fifties, and sixties aren't the sex-kitten seasons of your life, but that doesn't mean they can't bring you rich and fulfilling sensual experiences.

When to See Your Doctor

If you are dealing with feeling tired, frequently getting sick, and experiencing a loss of libido, I encourage you to make an appointment with your doctor for blood work, a medication review, and an open and honest conversation about what's going on in your life and what help you may need. Always remember: your doctor works for you and is in that medical office to support you. It is not a favor to fit you in, and your health concerns—even the ones you sometimes find difficult to talk about—deserve time and attention. Get comfortable being uncomfortable, and insist on the careful, thoughtful level of medical attention you deserve. If you're not finding that with your current practitioner, consider seeking out a functional medicine physician whose training is focused on whole-person health instead of a treat-and-release model. This comes back to the mentality we talked about in chapter 1: you are a matrix of miraculous energy, not a robot. Make sure your healthcare team treats you accordingly.

Here are the areas you may want to investigate with your physician:

Vitamin D: If you are not getting enough or are deficient, it can directly impact your energy. I urge you to get your vitamin D levels checked and ask your doctor if you should be taking a supplement.

Thyroid: The thyroid is a small, butterfly-shaped gland that impacts virtually all your other organs—regulating your metabolism, heartbeat, temperature, nervous system, cholesterol levels, menstrual cycles, and much, much more. It does all this by producing what's called "thyroid hormone" (TH), but sometimes things like stress, autoimmune disease, viral infections, toxins, nutritional deficiencies, and even pregnancy can cause your thyroid to start producing too much or too little TH.

Women are five to ten times more likely than men to develop thyroid issues. In fact, one in eight will develop a thyroid condition in her lifetime—and perhaps most importantly, up to 60% of those with thyroid disease don't know they have it.

Without considering the thyroid, we tend to attribute thyroid-related symptoms to other conditions. And this can go on for years, leading to lots of unnecessary suffering. Fortunately, there's growing awareness of the thyroid's critical role in health, which is why it's important to ask your doctor to get your levels checked.

Sexual health support: If you've been in the low sex drive season for too long, you're not alone. Hypoactive sexual desire disorder (a lack of desire that causes distress or interpersonal difficulty) is present in 8.9% of women ages eighteen to forty-four, 12.3% of ages forty-five to sixty-four, and 7.4% over sixty-five.

If your drop in sex drive is sudden, inexplicable to you, or inconsistent with what you've experienced in the past, consider scheduling a consultation with your ob-gyn or naturopathic physician. The fact is, less than half of patients with sexual problems seek help from or initiate discussions with physicians, and that number is far too low. Worse, I hear from many women who stop seeing their ob-gyn when they're done having kids—a choice that can leave them vulnerable to serious health issues in the long term. Consider making an appointment to have a checkup and talk about your low libido. I know it's uncomfortable, but there are prescription options you can explore. You may even already be on a medication that lowers your libido. Some common antidepressants like paroxetine (Paxil) and fluoxetine (Prozac, Sarafem) may cause a lower sex drive. As an alternative, bupropion (Wellbutrin SR, Wellbutrin XL), a different type of antidepressant, may be less disruptive. And statins lower serum testosterone in both men and women. These are just a few examples. Most doctors will work with you to find the right combination of medications so you don't have to sacrifice sex.

What's the Deal with Caffeine?

Truth be told, I only drink coffee once a week—and it's a collagen coffee. That's because I've never loved the jittery feeling I get after I drink caffeine. I also don't like to be what I call "fake awake." I do completely understand if you truly love the taste of coffee and what it means to you in life. However, it's important to know that there are a couple scientific reasons why your coffee habit may be making you more tired. Caffeine has been shown to block the adenosine receptors in the brain. Why does that matter? Adenosine causes fatigue and tells the brain when it's time to go to sleep. It also controls the amount of deep, restorative sleep you get.

Caffeine works because it blocks receptors in your brain from receiving adenosine, making you feel alert. But your body never stops producing adenosine, so once the caffeine wears off, you have a buildup of it that floods your body all at once, making you sleepy. Think of caffeine like a dam that holds back adenosine. Once removed, a flood of adenosine comes over you. Caffeine also has a half-life of five hours. Therefore, drinking coffee too close to bedtime will disrupt important restorative sleep, causing fatigue. Caffeine also indirectly releases adrenaline, which raises blood sugar. And after a rise in adrenaline and blood sugar comes . . . the crash. With a crash you'll probably reach for more caffeine. A vicious cycle.

Now if you love the taste of coffee and your morning latte is a daily moment of joy, I'd never take it away from you. I just advise you to stop drinking caffeine after 3:00 p.m. And if you're someone who strictly relies on coffee for energy, try matcha—a highly concentrated ground green tea that provides you with a big dose of phytonutrients—for a more "slow and steady" buzz. Think of matcha as super-tea—or, as some aficionados call it, "green tea on steroids." It's my go-to!

One last note about caffeine, and it's an important one: energy drinks are no friend of your gut, your actual energy level, or your immune system. They mask your fatigue by loading you with huge doses of caffeine. Many also contain taurine, which amplifies the effects of the caffeine. That's why these drinks frequently cause anxiety, "jitters," and insomnia. In addition, most energy drinks contain large amounts of either sugar or artificial sweeteners. The sugar-sweetened versions spike your blood glucose, raising your insulin levels and packing on belly fat, while the artificially-sweetened versions wreak havoc on the health of your gut bugs.

Perhaps worst of all, when the effects of an energy drink wear off, you'll crash—and that can tempt you to reach for a second drink or even a third one. Overdosing on energy drinks can raise your blood pressure, lead to cardiac arrhythmia, or, in rare cases, even cause cardiac arrest. More than twenty thousand people wind up in the emergency room annually due to the side effects of these drinks.

Foods and Supplements You Can Use

A Multivitamin

A multivitamin is a critical way to fill in nutrient gaps in your daily diet. This is especially true for immunity. A deficiency of single nutrients can alter the body's immune response. A regular multivitamin can help you avoid inadvertently missing out on important nutrients.

Immune- and Energy-Boosting Fruits and Veggies

Eating a diet of colorful fruits and vegetables rich in antioxidants is your best bet when you're looking to eat for immunity and energy. Everything in this food group is also full of fiber that will help nourish your microbiome, keep your cells clean, foster smooth digestion, and even keep your hormones in good regulation.

Spices

Many of your favorite spices offer far more than just a boost of flavor. Cinnamon, cumin, and oregano, for example, all contain antibacterial and antiviral properties.

Nuts and Sunflower Seeds

These snacks and salad toppers are rich in selenium, which does everything from reducing your cancer risk to fighting viruses to regulating your thyroid gland.

Oil of Oregano

This is another great go-to if you're battling a bug. Oil of oregano has powerful antibacterial, antiviral, and antifungal properties, and it can help you tackle all sorts of problems, including urinary tract infections, colds, flu, and even toenail fungus. You can buy oil of oregano in capsule form or opt for drops. If you choose drops, put a little bit in a vaporizer or diffuser, or add a small amount to a glass of water or juice. You can also combine one part oregano oil with three parts coconut or olive oil to make a healing skin cream. Oil of oregano is very powerful, so never use it straight, either internally or on your skin. Also, do a "spot test" with a tiny amount to make sure you're not allergic to it. One important caution: Do *not* use oil of oregano either orally or topically if you are pregnant or nursing.

Zinc-Rich Foods

Foods in this category, including pumpkin seeds, beef and other dark meats, crab, turkey, lobster, chicken, and beef liver are truly something to "zinc" about because they're a two-for-one on the energy-libido front. Your immune system needs zinc to function optimally, and it appears to work in two ways: by interfering with a virus's ability to reproduce and by blocking its ability to attach to cell membranes.

But that's not all. When studied in an intervention group of women, zinc supplementation significantly improved sexual desire, arousal, orgasm, satisfaction, and vaginal moisture, and decreased pain during intercourse.

The ultimate zinc-rich food is one that's synonymous with arousal: *oysters.* Turns out there's some hard science behind this legendary aphrodisiac.

If none of the zinc-containing foods are part of your diet, you can also get this nutrient in the form of a supplement.

Vitamin D

You'll find a lot of reasons to consider a vitamin D supplement in this book, and here is another: vitamin D deficiency is associated with abnormal female sexual functioning. Given sufficient sunlight, the body can synthesize vitamin D, and foods that are high in this essential vitamin include cod liver oil, salmon, sardines, and egg yolks.

Fiber

Long story short (and yes, I know this is a story I tell often, but only because it is so very important): fiber balances hormones. Soluble fiber, such as the kind found in fruits, helps to remove excess estrogen from your body.

Pick-Me-Up Bone Broth

This fast and simple version of egg drop soup will fortify you and lift your spirits. It's a sense of renewed energy in a mug.

PREP TIME: 5 min.

COOK TIME: 3 min. and 10 min. wait time

YIELD: 1 serving

1 cup Chicken Bone Broth (page 272) or store-bought, plus more as needed

1 ($^{1}/_{2}$- to 1-inch) piece peeled fresh ginger

1 small garlic clove, smashed

1 large egg, whisked

1 handful of spinach, chopped

1 to 2 button or cremini mushrooms, thinly sliced, optional

Pinch of Celtic sea or pink Himalayan salt, or coconut aminos

Pinch of freshly ground black pepper

In a small saucepan over medium-high heat, add the bone broth, ginger, and garlic and bring to a boil. Slowly pour in the egg, whisking constantly. Add the spinach and mushrooms, cover, turn off the heat, and steep for about 10 minutes to let flavors meld. Season with the salt and pepper.

Pot of Gold: Creamy Broccoli Soup with Ginger

I love creamy soups, and I like to keep my cooking quick and easy whenever I can. This soup will give you a little boost because of the energizing and immune-supporting ingredients that are nutrient rich. It's always been one of my go-to favorites, and adding the pepitas really rounds out the flavor. It keeps well in the refrigerator (if there are any leftovers) and easily reheats.

PREP TIME: 15 min.
COOK TIME: 25 min.
YIELD: 4 to 6 servings

2 tablespoons ghee

1 medium onion, diced

2 garlic cloves, minced

1 quart (4 cups) Chicken Bone Broth (page 272) or store-bought

1 cup unsweetened full-fat coconut milk (from a can)

4 cups broccoli florets

1 (1-inch) piece peeled fresh ginger, grated

1 teaspoon Celtic sea or pink Himalayan salt

$^1/_2$ teaspoon freshly ground black pepper

$^1/_2$ cup raw pepitas, finely ground

$^1/_2$ cup toasted whole pepitas, for garnish, optional

Ground nutmeg, for garnish, optional

In a large stockpot over medium-high heat, melt the ghee. Add the onion, reduce heat to medium, and sauté for 6 to 8 minutes to soften. Add the garlic and sauté for another minute. Increase the heat to medium-high, add the bone broth, coconut milk, broccoli, ginger, salt, and pepper. When the soup begins to simmer, reduce the heat to medium-low and simmer for 15 to 20 minutes or until the broccoli is tender. Add the ground pepitas. Purée the soup with a hand-held immersion blender, blender, or food processor until smooth and creamy (see Notes). Serve garnished with the toasted pepitas and a pinch of nutmeg (if using).

Key ingredients for vitality and immune support: bone broth, garlic, broccoli, ginger, pepitas

NOTES
The easiest way to grind pepitas is in a coffee grinder, but you can use a food processor.

If you use a blender or food processor for the soup, process in batches, covering the top with a clean kitchen towel to avoid getting burned.

Pot of Gold: Oyster Stew

There are stories throughout history about oysters as an aphrodisiac. Casanova, an eighteenth-century Italian intellectual, became famous for his erotic memoir *The Story of My Life*, in which he attributed his raging libido to eating fifty oysters for breakfast every day. Fact or fiction? Either way, that's too much! My oyster stew, on the other hand, is a just-right pick-me-up on a chilly day—and a perfect dish to share with somebody you'd like to snuggle up with after dinner.

PREP TIME: 20 min.
COOK TIME: 20 min.
YIELD: 4 to 5 servings

3 tablespoons ghee or pasture-raised butter

2 leeks (white parts only), thinly sliced

3 celery stalks, diced

1 garlic clove, minced

$1/_2$ teaspoon dried or 1 teaspoon minced fresh thyme leaves

1 quart (4 cups) Chicken (page 272) or Fish Bone Broth (page 275) or store-bought

1 dried bay leaf

1 large waxy potato, peeled and cut into $1/_2$-inch cubes

1 (14-ounce) can full-fat coconut milk

1 tablespoon coarsely chopped flat-leaf parsley, plus more for garnishing, optional

$1/_2$ teaspoon Celtic sea or Pink Himalayan salt

$1/_2$ teaspoon freshly ground black pepper

$1^1/_2$ pints (three 8-ounce jars) refrigerated shucked oysters (see Notes)

In a stockpot over medium heat, melt the ghee and add the leeks and celery. Sauté for 7 to 8 minutes. Add the garlic and thyme and sauté for another minute. Add the bone broth and bay leaf, increase the heat to medium-high, and bring to a low boil. Add the potatoes, reduce the heat to medium, and simmer for 12 to 15 minutes or until just fork tender. Add the coconut milk, parsley, salt, and pepper, and bring back to a simmer. Add the oysters and continue to simmer just until the edges curl, about 3 minutes (overcooking will make them tough). Remove the bay leaf before serving and garnish with the parsley (if using).

Key ingredients for energy and libido boost: bone broth, garlic, oysters, potato, parsley

NOTES

This is not meant to be a thick soup like New England clam chowder. It's more like a Southern-style oyster stew with a buttery broth.

For the oysters, check the jar to see how they are packed. If they are packed in water, you may want to rinse them. If they are packed in liqueur, this means they are packed in the juice that was in the shell when they were shucked. This is common in higher-quality products, and you can add some or all of it to the stew.

Jars of smaller oysters may have as many as 30 per pint. Jars of medium oysters average 16 to 18 per pint. If the oysters are too large, cut them into smaller pieces. A large oyster is too big to eat in one bite.

Pot of Gold: Portuguese Sausage, Kale, and Potato Soup (Caldo Verde)

The first time I enjoyed this soup, I was in a cozy oceanside restaurant on a blustery fall day. It sounded interesting so I tried it—and loved it so much I had to create a recipe to emulate those warm and smoky flavors. Caldo verde, translated as "green soup" because of the kale, is a homey, rustic, and comforting soup from Spain. Traditionally chorizo, a spicy cured pork sausage, is used in place of the kielbasa, and you can use it if you prefer. Just check the ingredients for sugar and nitrates. Because chorizo contains vinegar, I prefer the mellower flavor of kielbasa.

PREP TIME: 15 min.
COOK TIME: 35 min.
YIELD: 6 to 8 servings

2 tablespoons avocado oil

1 pound natural uncured turkey kielbasa, cut into $3/4$-inch rounds

1 medium onion, diced

2 to 3 garlic cloves, minced

2 quarts (8 cups) Chicken Bone Broth (page 272) or store-bought

1 bunch of kale, cut in $1/2$-inch ribbons (stems and center veins removed; about 2 cups)

$1/2$ teaspoon Celtic sea or pink Himalayan salt

$1/2$ teaspoon freshly ground black pepper

$3/4$ pound (about 4 medium) waxy potatoes, diced into $1/2$-inch cubes (see Note)

Crushed red pepper flakes, for serving

In a large stockpot over medium-high heat, add the oil and kielbasa and sauté for 3 to 4 minutes. Add the onion and sauté for another 3 to 4 minutes to soften the onion. Add the garlic and sauté for another minute. Add the bone broth, kale, salt, and pepper. Cover and cook for about 5 minutes until the kale begins to soften. Add the potatoes. Simmer, covered, for about 15 minutes or until the potatoes are fork tender. Serve garnished with the red pepper flakes.

Key ingredients for vitality and immune support: bone broth, garlic, kale

NOTE

Waxy potatoes have a thin, papery skin that can be easily scratched off with your fingernail. Red potatoes, new potatoes, Yukon gold potatoes, and fingerling potatoes are all types of waxy potatoes. They have a lower starch content, and given their waxy nature, they hold their shape well as they cook. In contrast, starchy potatoes, such as russets, will fall apart when cooked.

Slow-Cooker Turkey and Sweet Potato Stew

Put this together in the morning, dash off to enjoy your day, and come home to a hearty, satisfying dinner. I promise you'll smile when you walk in the door and smell the scrumptious aroma coming from your kitchen. Turkey isn't just for Thanksgiving, and yet it's only served once or twice a year in many households. I find turkey to be a welcome change from chicken (though chicken is also delicious in this recipe). Enjoy this easy one-pot meal on a chilly evening.

PREP TIME: 20 min.

COOK TIME: 4 hrs. on high or 6 hrs. on low

YIELD: 4 to 6 servings

1 pound skinless turkey or chicken breasts or thighs (see Notes)

2 sweet potatoes, peeled and cut into 2-inch cubes (about 14 ounces)

3 carrots, cut into rounds

1 small onion, sliced

2 garlic cloves, smashed

$1/2$ teaspoon ground sage or $3/4$ teaspoon rubbed sage (see Notes)

1 teaspoon dried thyme

Pinch of ground cinnamon

$1^1/_2$ quarts (6 cups) Chicken Bone Broth (page 272) or store-bought

2 teaspoons Celtic sea or pink Himalayan salt

1 teaspoon freshly ground black pepper

In a 6- to 8-quart slow cooker, add all the ingredients. Cover and cook on high for 4 hours or on low for 6 hours. Remove the turkey and shred into 1-inch pieces with two forks, return to the pot, and serve.

Key ingredients for vitality and immune support: bone broth, sweet potatoes, garlic, cinnamon

NOTES

You can use all white-meat turkey or chicken, but using some dark meat will add an extra depth of flavor. Slow cooking results in incredibly tender meat.

Ground sage is more concentrated than rubbed sage, and they work equally well.

If you'd like a creamy stew, 30 minutes before it's done, remove about half the sweet potatoes and carrots along with some of the juices and purée in a blender or food processor with $1/2$ cup or more full-fat coconut milk (make sure to cover the top with a clean kitchen towel to avoid getting burned). Return the mixture to the slow cooker and stir.

Italian Frittata with Sausage, Roasted Red Peppers, and Mushrooms

A frittata is a baked egg dish enriched with meat and/or vegetables. If you haven't made one in the past, you'll find this remarkably simple, and the final dish is light and fluffy. Slice it as you would a pie, add a fresh green salad, and dinner is on the table. It is also great for breakfast or lunch. It stores well in the refrigerator, reheats quickly in the microwave, and makes a great grab-and-go meal.

PREP TIME: 15 min.
COOK TIME: 30 min.
YIELD: 4 to 5 servings

3 tablespoons ghee or avocado oil, divided

$^1/_2$ pound button or cremini mushrooms, sliced (about 2$^1/_2$ cups)

1 small onion, diced

1 pound natural nitrate-, gluten-, and sugar-free Italian turkey sausage, sliced or removed from casing

$^3/_4$ cup drained and dried jarred roasted red peppers, diced or cut into strips

8 large eggs

1$^1/_2$ teaspoons Italian seasoning

$^1/_2$ teaspoon Celtic sea or pink Himalayan salt

$^1/_4$ teaspoon freshly ground black pepper

$^1/_8$ to $^1/_4$ teaspoon crushed red pepper flakes

Pinch of garlic powder

Place an oven rack in the center of the oven and preheat it to 350°F.

In an oven-proof skillet, such as cast iron (see Note), over medium-high heat, melt 2 tablespoons of the ghee. Add the mushrooms and sauté for 7 to 8 minutes or until they start to turn golden. If there is liquid in the pan, continue to cook until the liquid has evaporated. Add the onions and sauté for 4 to 5 minutes. Remove the mushroom mixture from pan and set aside. Add the remaining 1 tablespoon ghee and the sausage to the pan and sauté for about 5 minutes until done. Return the mushroom mixture to the pan and stir in the roasted red peppers.

In a large bowl, whisk the eggs with the Italian seasoning, salt, pepper, red pepper flakes, and garlic powder. Pour the egg mixture into the pan and use a fork to evenly distribute it over the sausage mixture. Cook for 1 to 2 minutes until the eggs begin to firm.

Transfer the pan to the oven and bake, uncovered, for about 20 minutes or until the center has puffed up and the frittata is set. Test by inserting a knife into the center.

Key ingredients for vitality and immune support: garlic, mushrooms, eggs, red peppers, crushed red pepper flakes

———

NOTE

If you don't have an oven-proof skillet, transfer the sausage mixture to a baking dish. In a large bowl, whisk the eggs with the Italian seasoning, salt, pepper, and red pepper flakes, and pour the eggs over the sausage mixture. Bake, uncovered, for about 20 minutes.

Sweet Potato Mash with Indian Spices

There is a warmth and depth to Indian spices that I have always enjoyed. I feel satisfied after an Indian meal. If you enjoy these aromatic spices as much as I do, I'm certain you'll love this sweet potato dish. The oven does most of the work; you just need to warm the ghee and spices. It's a great accompaniment to most broiled or grilled meats and is especially delicious in the fall and winter when there's a chill in the air.

PREP TIME: 10 min.

COOK TIME: 40 to 50 min.

YIELD: 4 to 6 servings

2 pounds sweet potatoes, scrubbed

3 tablespoons ghee

$^1/_2$ teaspoon ground coriander

$^1/_2$ teaspoon ground cumin

$^1/_2$ teaspoon ground turmeric

$^1/_2$ teaspoon ground ginger

$^1/_4$ teaspoon ground cinnamon

$^1/_8$ teaspoon ground cayenne pepper, optional

1 teaspoon Celtic sea or pink Himalayan salt

$^1/_2$ teaspoon freshly ground black pepper

2 tablespoons freshly squeezed lime juice (from about 1 lime)

$^1/_4$ to $^1/_2$ cup Chicken Bone Broth (page 272) or store-bought

3 tablespoons coarsely chopped fresh cilantro (discard stems), plus more for garnish, optional

Place an oven rack in the center of the oven and preheat it to 425°F. Line a baking sheet with parchment paper or foil.

Poke each potato four or five times with a fork to release steam while roasting. Place the sweet potatoes onto the prepared baking sheet (do not wrap them in foil). Bake for 40 to 50 minutes or until very soft. Test them with a knife—they should be creamy on the inside.

Meanwhile, in a small sauté pan over low heat, melt the ghee. Stir in the coriander, cumin, turmeric, ginger, cinnamon, and cayenne pepper (if using). Warm for 1 to 2 minutes or until the spices become fragrant. Add the salt and pepper and set aside until the sweet potatoes are done baking.

When the sweet potatoes are ready, rewarm the spice mixture over low heat. Scrape the insides of the sweet potatoes into a bowl and pour the spice mixture, the lime juice, bone broth, and cilantro over the potatoes and mash. Garnish with additional cilantro (if using).

Key ingredients for vitality and immunity support: sweet potatoes, turmeric, bone broth, ginger; the warm spices also have a soothing and comforting effect

---

NOTES

If you are a lover of curry, you can add $^1/_2$ teaspoon or more curry powder to the spice mix.

If you want the dish to have more moisture, add additional bone broth.

Chocolate Bark with Pistachios and Oranges

I'm not even sure if it's humanly possible not to love dark chocolate. We can thank the Maya and Aztecs for introducing it to the rest of the world. Once only enjoyed by the elite, we have it at our fingertips whenever the craving arises now. Dark chocolate increases serotonin levels and acts as a mild stimulant, increasing our feel-good endorphins. Great for a boost of energy, and a great dessert to enjoy with a hot date.

PREP TIME: 30 min.
YIELD: About 1¹/₄ pounds

1 medium navel orange

3 tablespoons coconut sugar

¹/₂ to 1 teaspoon pure orange extract or 1 tablespoon orange liqueur, optional

16 ounces dark or bittersweet stevia-sweetened chocolate, at least 72% dark

1 cup salted roasted pistachios, very roughly chopped

Line a baking sheet with parchment paper and draw a square about 10 × 10 inches. Flip the paper over onto the baking sheet to create a template for spreading the chocolate.

Using a mandolin or a very sharp knife, slice the orange into very thin rounds, then cut in half. In a saucepan over medium-high heat, add 1 cup of water, the coconut sugar, and orange extract (if using). Bring to a boil and stir to dissolve the sugar. Add the orange slices and reduce the heat to medium-low. Gently simmer for 15 to 20 minutes or until most of the liquid has evaporated and the oranges are in a thick syrup. Remove the oranges from pan and spread them out in a single layer on waxed or parchment paper to cool.

In a double boiler or a heatproof bowl set over a saucepan of simmering water, melt the chocolate (make sure the water doesn't touch the bottom of the bowl). Be careful not to get any water in the chocolate or it will seize.

Pour the chocolate onto the prepared parchment paper, keeping it within the stencil. Place the orange slices randomly over the chocolate and then sprinkle with the pistachios. Set aside for several hours until firm, but don't refrigerate. When fully cooled, break or slice the bark into pieces and serve at room temperature. Store between layers of waxed or parchment paper in a sealed container, in a cool, dry place.

Key ingredients for energy and libido: dark chocolate, pistachios

NOTES

If you have any orange slices with a bit of syrup left over, you can use them to garnish or baste chicken or pork.

You can substitute other nuts in this recipe.

Chapter 10

Soothe Yourself:
What's Your Stress Type?

I n every life, a little rain must fall. And sorrow. And *stress*. Stress can come from heartbreak, from life's relentless demands, and can sometimes arise out of opportunities that bring unexpected pressures.

I don't know a soul—even among women with health and beauty who appear to have it all—who glides through life without anything going wrong. The beautiful woman with that je ne sais quoi may *look* like everything is perfect, but I promise you, she, too, suffers. Hardships may not get meted out to all of us in equal measure, but everybody has hurts, traumas, and daily pressures. The truth of the matter is that over the twenty years I was working in clinical practice, more than two thirds of the patients I saw had levels of stress that were negatively impacting their health, their looks, or their mental outlooks.

Stress is never going to go away completely. But you can learn to halt its downward spiral—and that starts by knowing your stress type. In my clinical practice, I could usually categorize people who were super stressed into one of three types. Helping patients learn their type clued us in to what steps to take next. Gaining awareness of how you're feeling—and how you're dealing—is the key to getting stress troubles under control.

Is it a teensy bit nineties *Cosmo* to include a quiz here? You got me. But if you're anything like me, you never let one of those quizzes pass you by, because we are all constantly looking for answers. I can't think of an area where those answers matter more than in helping us learn how to dial down the impact of stress on our lives.

QUESTION 1: When you're put in a stressful situation, are you most likely to:
   A. Step up and take charge. The adrenaline drives you.
   B. Become paralyzed and take no action, not unlike a deer in headlights.
   C. Focus on something else, anything but the situation at hand.

QUESTION 2: When you're in a high state of stress, what are you most likely to experience physically?
   A. Adrenaline: the big jolt of *oomph* that helps you get stuff done in a hurry.
   B. Nausea or cramps: high stress equals instant illness.
   C. Nothing. You go numb.

QUESTION 3: Describe your eating habits when you're stressed.
   A. Too busy to eat.
   B. Sometimes you're too sick to your stomach to eat; other times you're looking for comfort food.
   C. Likely to eat mindlessly to distract yourself or numb the stress.

QUESTION 4: What best describes your sleeping habits when you're stressed?
   A. You stay up late and wake up early. Sleep is your last priority.
   B. You just want to crawl into bed. Stress takes away your energy.
   C. Your sleep is rarely disrupted by stress.

QUESTION 5: Which of the following actions help you calm your stress?

    A. Make a to-do list.

    B. Write in a journal.

    C. Watch television.

If you answered mostly A's, you're a Short-Term Stress Type

We all have short-term pressures and shake-ups that impact our lives. Maybe your kid just announced a big science project is due *tomorrow*—and even though you've been teaching accountability since he could walk, this somehow feels like *your* problem. Maybe you've got a big meeting or evaluation coming up at work. Maybe you're in the middle of a spat with a friend or partner. Maybe you're helping someone get through a temporary illness. When these things happen, you know what to do: buckle up and do the work. The trouble is that this stress type is more likely to forego sleep and rely on things like stimulants to keep the adrenaline pumping until the stress passes. You will benefit most if you focus on stamina-care.

If you answered mostly B's, you're a Chronic Stress Type

Long-term, or chronic, stress is a different challenge. It happens when you can't ever see the light at the end of the tunnel; sometimes you're in that state for so long you stop even looking for the light. In terms of your health, chronic stress is no different than eating fast food every single day. That's how much it inflames and distorts your body and mind.

When ongoing stress keeps that cortisol flowing, you risk suffering from a raft of unpleasant and difficult symptoms, among them:

Muscle tension	*Chronic fatigue*
Pain	*Poor sleep*

Food cravings

Loss of motivation

A sense of isolation

Depression

Mood swings

Weight gain

Acne, eczema, and other skin issues

See what I mean? Like eating fast food every day.

Perhaps worse than any of these symptoms is the fact that, if you get into a stress spiral, it can wreak havoc on all your healthy habits.

If you answered mostly C's, you're an Avoiding Stress Type

You'd rather completely avoid and distract yourself from stress than face it head on or let it knock you off balance. However, in the attempt to avoid stress, you may have developed some unhealthy coping mechanisms that throw you off balance in other ways.

When I see people with Chronic and Avoiding Stress Types, I worry a lot about cortisol. Cortisol is released in response to stress or fear as part of the body's fight or flight response. That's why this hormone is commonly called the "stress hormone," or as I like to call it, "the belly-fat hormone." Cortisol performs critical functions in the body, including helping to manage your metabolism, regulating your blood pressure and sugar levels, keeping your sleep cycle on track, and regulating your stress responses.

Because it plays a critical role in so many vital systems that impact how you're feeling and how you're doing, when cortisol gets out of whack—well, it unleashes a storm of troubles that can impact nearly every facet of your health and wellness. Just re-read the list above if you need a reminder of the many ways stress impacts you.

I'm an ardent proponent of the power of momentum, but the kind of momentum stress brings to your life is the worst, sinking you lower and lower. It can leave you vulnerable to neglecting your healthy lifestyle—by making damaging choices like drinking too much, exercising too little, indulging in nutritionally empty foods, or skimping on sleep. Which is why, in addition to stamina-care (which is good for everyone), these two types will really benefit from focusing on diet and sleep as well.

A Time to Be Gentle

What I've learned—sometimes the hard way—is that the *worst* time to force a workout, to literally go the extra mile, is when you are struggling with chronic stress. Having a bad or stressful day? Sure, a vigorous workout can sometimes turn a bad day around, revving up your metabolism and getting your happy hormones flowing.

But if you've gone weeks or even months when stress is persistent, you don't need to tax your body ever further. It's one thing to be a cadet in military training. If you are, then you can and should expect that a workout will be piled on top of your already stressful day! *That* kind of workout is part of a meticulously planned (though admittedly harsh) program to build and train you *up* so you know you can perform in an emergency situation. But if you're just living your day-to-day life, persistent stress is not part of a program to build you up. Instead, you're more likely in the middle of a long process of breaking down.

Think about what you'd tell a friend who's feeling crushed by a high-pressure job, a grinding commute, family drama, health worries, or any other combination of major stressors that are taking a toll. Would you look into her tired, dark, circle-rimmed eyes and tell her to get her butt to the gym and *push on through, dammit?*

Or would you suggest she take a walk in the sun? Or join you for a low-impact yoga class? Or ride her bike through the park? I know you've got a good heart, and I'm positive you'd choose a form of movement that would help bring this woman back to center. We need to build her up gently.

Look, it's a fact that exercise is a cure-all for many physical and mental health problems. After sleep and nutrition, it is the next most powerful tool at your disposal to combat stress. In terms of straight-up neurochemistry, it gets to the heart of the problem—reducing your levels of cortisol while at the same time stimulating production of endorphins that offer the body a natural pick-me-up. Equally important, exercise improves the flow of oxygen to all your cells, and that helps them heal from the damage excess cortisol, and the lack of sleep that often accompanies it, does.

But when you are stressed out, you have a particular obligation to be gentle and kind with yourself. Over the years, I've met far too many people who exercise in ways that look an awful lot like trying to *punish* themselves out of their stress—and it simply does not work.

What does work? Engage in slow movement exercises like yoga, Tai Chi, walking, or swimming. If you can possibly manage it, do them outside where you can get the extra benefit of sunlight and fresh air. Shoot for twenty to thirty minutes of gentle activity twice a day. When you have to make-do with less, accept it and try again tomorrow.

Most important, while you're spending that time, ask yourself the one question that matters most: is this activity breaking me down, or is it building me up?

Stress Eating

We've all been there. A lot of us were there *frequently* during the pandemic. Stress eating is real, and it's important to know that it's not so much a problem as it is a symptom. A symptom of stress.

I can't think of many people who don't suffer from some degree of stress eating. Take the classic children's book *The Very Hungry Caterpillar*. It's a story meant to be about an evolution that is just as much a story about stress eating. That little caterpillar ate "one piece of chocolate cake, one ice-cream cone, one pickle, one slice of Swiss cheese, one slice of salami, one lollipop, one piece of cherry pie, one sausage, one cupcake, and one slice of watermelon"—all on a Saturday afternoon. And what happened? He had a tummy ache. And what made him feel better?

A green leaf. Eric Carle seems to have known about gut health way before many of us nutrition professionals did.

Let's get real about how the foods we emotionally eat play into that stress spiral. Caffeine and processed sugar (including simple carbs like crackers and breads that your body almost instantly turns to sugar) can add *to* the stress you're experiencing because of other aggravations. In fact, sugar is one of the building blocks of stress hormones. Consuming it when you're already stressed can kick off a relentless cycle of cravings and crashes and crashes and cravings. And at night, the caffeine and sugar that kept you on this daytime roller coaster can also interfere with your ability to get the sleep you desperately need.

Unfortunately, there are no foods that simply and instantly turn off stress, but there are plenty of options that can help bring your body and mind back to a quiet balance. Some of these are effective because they boost your serotonin levels, providing a calming effect on the chemical levels in your brain. These are "comfort foods" in the truest sense of the term. Incorporating some or all of these foods into your regular meal plans can also lower your blood pressure and boost your immune system. Adding these nutrient-rich options to your regular diet can give you a giant edge on stress.

Foods You Can Use

Bone Broth

But of course!

Bone broth is my secret weapon for all kinds of nutritional healing, but especially for stress. Much more than just a broth or soup, it is one of the world's oldest and most powerful medicinal foods. And because it supports health at a cellular level, I turn to this nutrient-rich elixir multiple times a day when I'm under stress. In fact, it is one of the rituals I adhere to most closely when I'm feeling pressure. Sipping on it at my first meal of the day helps set the tone for how I'll eat for the next several hours. Enjoying it as a midday snack helps fill me up so I eat less throughout the day. And sipping a mug of bone broth at the end of a harried day relaxes and centers me.

In reality, bone broth offers a trifecta of antidotes to stress: It bathes your system in alkaline minerals that reduce the impacts of stress-induced acidity. It helps you feel full so you don't get crushed by the cravings stress creates. And it helps heal your gut with its powerful liquid collagen. Plus, it's a small, simple step toward wellness during those times when a big win feels impossible to find.

Almonds

If you don't already keep almonds around as a snack, it's time to add them to your pantry. Almonds provide a boost of energy and keep you satisfied when you feel hunger or cravings arise. They're a rich source of vitamin E, which supports a healthy immune system, and also of B vitamins, which may help you fight spells of anxiety and depression. Since they're a great natural source of both melatonin and magnesium, which provide sleep support, almonds are an ideal inclusion to your last meal or snack of the day.

Artichokes

Artichokes are a great source of a wide spectrum of vitamins and minerals, including magnesium, potassium, and vitamin C. This oddest looking of vegetables is also an outstanding source of fiber and those prebiotics we talked about in chapter 7. That combo makes them a strong ally of gut health—and a healthy gut is essential to soothing stress.

Avocados

Avocados always make the cut on my list of superfoods, and when it comes to helping you manage stress, they do so on multiple levels. These green beauties are rich in fiber, healthy fats, vitamins, and minerals— and studies show they can help protect you against high blood sugar levels and high blood pressure. Plus, half an avocado is a higher source of potassium than a banana. All that potassium helps to relax your blood vessels.

The best thing about avocados, of course, is that they're delicious. If you're looking for an easy, tasty way to spruce up a salad or omelet, an avocado with a spritz of lemon or a sprinkle of salt is your answer.

Butternut Squash

One of the most frustrating aspects of chronic stress is that it drives cravings for sweets. Enter this palate-pleasing squash—a nutrient-rich, high-fiber energy carb that has *just enough* sweetness to take the edge off those sometimes overwhelming urges to indulge. This is a comfort food that can soothe your taste buds without wrecking your healthful diet—plus it's an outstanding source of potassium, which can keep your blood vessels relaxed. This squash is delicious roasted with a little coconut oil and pink Himalayan salt, but for a dish that's a true balm for stress, try my Butternut-Apple Soup with Warming Spices (page 230). It's an elixir that combines the benefits of this yummy winter squash with the powerful nutrition of bone broth.

Citrus Fruits and Berries

Full of vitamin C, oranges are an ideal stress-relieving food. They can naturally lower stress hormone levels and boost your immune system. Not sold? That vitamin C also supports your body's production of collagen—and that means healthy, radiant skin and fabulous anti-aging benefits! Research has shown this most delicious of stress-relief foods can also help lower cortisol and blood pressure levels.

Eggs

Eggs are nature's most neatly packaged nutrient bomb. They're loaded with protein, vitamins, and minerals. One of the lesser-known nutrients they're rich in is *choline*, which boosts nervous-system health. A healthy nervous system equals a body and mind that are able to cope with stress.

Raw, Crunchy Vegetables

A study of over four hundred young adults in New Zealand compared intakes of raw versus cooked vegetables and found that eating raw was correlated with reduced symptoms of depression, higher life satisfaction, better mood, and higher levels of what respondents called "flourishing."

You gotta love a study that's trying to get at the essence of flourishing.

Now I'm all for eating veggies in *any* form you enjoy—the nutritional benefits are endless—so why the recommendation for raw varieties in particular? A lot of people hold tension in their jaw (hence expressions like "jaws clenched" and "biting my tongue" when we talk about how we feel in stressful situations). Crunching on veggies gives this tension-holding part of you a job to do that can help you let some of that stress go. Here's my advice: Embrace raw veggies in their simplest forms whenever you can. One of my favorite snacks on a hot day is a fresh cucumber. Slice it up or quarter it if you like, or just eat it like a candy bar!

And of all the culinary fads in the new millennium that have made my life easier, nothing can hold a candle to the *chopped salad*. Here, finally, is a way for us to eat and *enjoy* many of those vegetables that kids have been stuffing into heat registers for a hundred years. Brussels sprouts, zucchini, celery root, kale, baby artichoke, asparagus—all of them are fabulous shaved or shredded and tossed together with olive oil and vinegar or your favorite dressing.

Unclench that jaw and start nibbling on your veggies. They can truly help you wind your stress levels down.

Salmon and Tuna

These nutrient-rich foods contain omega-3 fatty acids that help curb stress hormone levels and support brain health, plus high-quality protein to help keep your blood sugar on an even keel. Consistent fatty fish consumption has so many health benefits, I make it a priority in my own diet and recommend it to everyone I meet. Plus it's a cinch to put together a healthy meal in minutes when fish is your protein source. You can sauté, bake, broil, or grill and use any favorite spice. Add half an avocado and a hearty serving of any veggie, and you've got yourself a power breakfast, lunch, or dinner.

Spinach

Spinach deserves a special shout-out over the other veggies. When you battle stress and the tension headaches that can come with it, this one food can make a world of difference. Chronic stress depletes your body of magnesium, and since that's the very mineral that modulates your stress response, this can quickly become a debilitating cycle of low magnesium, high stress, low magnesium. Research tells us increasing magnesium can ease stress and anxiety, and just one cup of spinach can boost your magnesium levels to restore balance and prevent headaches. Spinach is so easy to mix into anything you're having already—throw a handful into a salad, cook it in your eggs, bake it in a casserole, quickly wilt it into a cup of bone broth, or add it to any sautéed dish. I strongly recommend incorporating a cup of it into your diet as many days as possible.

Supplements

There are a number of nutritional supplements that can help your body cope with stress. If you take prescription medications, check with your doctor before adding anything new to your regimen.

- Omega-3: The good fairy of fatty acids waves her wand when it comes to stress. Omega-3 supplements have been shown to reduce cortisol levels both during and after stressful events. They also reduce levels of an inflammatory protein at the same time. This points toward less harm being done to the body during stressful events (read: less *aging*). Fatty fish, oysters, flax seeds, chia seeds, and walnuts are all great dietary sources.
- Vitamin C: One of the things that often goes unrecognized when we talk about stress is that, in addition to prepping you for fight or flight, your stress response also reduces immune function. Studies on both animals and people tell us that vitamin C supplementation can help on both counts. It's been shown to reduce the levels of stress hormones in the bloodstream and lift the levels of your body's antibodies to guard against systemic infection. Citrus fruits, peppers, berries, tomatoes, potatoes, and cruciferous vegetables like broccoli and cabbage are all great dietary sources.
- Vitamin E: You likely know vitamin E as a balm for the *outside* of your body because it's in so many moisturizing products. But on the inside, vitamin E is also a soothing force. There's even some evidence from animal studies that anxiety-like behavior can be a *symptom* of vitamin E deficiency. The upshot of this is that when your body is under stress, it gobbles up vitamin E. A little extra dose of this nutrient can help

keep you balanced. Leafy greens, pumpkin, almonds, peanuts, aspara- gus, avocados, and mangoes are all great dietary sources.

- Potassium: An estimated 98% of Americans don't get enough potas- sium in their diets. *98%?!* In addition to helping keep your blood ves- sels relaxed, this nutrient regulates fluid levels throughout the body to keep your cells healthy, and it helps keep your blood pressure in check as a balance to pressure-raising sodium. Besides the banana (every- body's favorite gold star potassium source), sweet potatoes, squash, spinach, avocados, mushrooms, cucumbers, and broccoli are all great dietary sources.

- Magnesium: When you get stressed out, your magnesium level is often the first thing to drop. As a relaxing alternative to pills and diet changes, you can replenish this essential mineral by adding one cup of Epsom salts to your bath. Tell your family it's doctor's orders, and enjoy a fif- teen-minute soak to get that magnesium level back up where it be- longs. Pumpkin seeds, spinach, nuts (especially almonds and cashews), yogurt, avocados, and edamame are all great dietary sources.

- Ashwagandha: For thousands of years, before you and I lived with the luxury of fully stocked pharmacies and medicine cabinets, ancient cul- tures were using substances found in nature to combat fatigue, soothe stress, and ease anxiety. As a group, we call these supplements adaptogens—plants that help bring our systems back into balance. Ashwagandha is one of these. The roots of this evergreen shrub from India have been used in Ayurvedic medicine for thousands of years. A small but growing body of research shows it can help lower cortisol levels, moderate stress symptoms, and reduce stress-related weight gain. The downside of this supplement is that it has a bitter taste. For that reason, if you're going to give it a trial run, you may want to choose a capsule or gummy form rather than a powder.

Tea Up at Bedtime

For thousands of years, people have been drinking tea in all its forms—white, black, green, herbal, and more—believing it has healing powers. In recent years, research is starting to bear out what we've long suspected: the tea in your mug is, in fact, a center of calm in a storm.

In one study, for example, researchers weaned their subjects off both coffee and tea for four weeks. After that, one group drank tea every day for six weeks, while the other consumed a placebo drink. When researchers brought these subjects into a lab and had them perform challenging tasks that universally raised their blood pressure, heart rate, and stress levels, their cortisol levels were measured before and after. The tea drinkers' cortisol levels were lower than their placebo-drinking peers. Not only that, but they knew it. They rated themselves as more relaxed.

One of the key reasons tea eases stress is the L-theanine it contains. This amino acid, even isolated from the cuppa, has been shown to reduce stress and anxiety in people who are struggling with either. If you want to maximize your intake, black tea contains the most L-theanine, but other teas have it in lower levels.

The upshot of the research (not to mention millions of real-life users' devotion over millennia) is that a cup of tea really is a powerful tool for stress reduction. If you need more convincing, set a boundary that your one cup of tea equals ten minutes of quiet time to relax and reflect. The simple act of starting your nightly shutdown with a few minutes of quiet sipping from a warm mug sets the stage for sleep.

Lay Your Burden Down

As a mere human, you need sleep to survive. Every day, we have to accept this fact again. And for as long as people have been talking about bedtime, they've been marking it as a moment to unburden themselves and find some peace—even if only for a little while.

Go with this flow. Choose a favorite quote or ritual to punctuate the turning point from your day to your night. It could be the serenity prayer or a favorite poem, *Goodnight Moon* or a proverb (I'm partial to the Irish one that says, "A good laugh and a long sleep are the two best cures for anything"). Whatever you choose, make it your bedtime mantra—a point when you relinquish everything you're carrying until morning.

While you're sleeping, your cortisol levels will reset, your body will soothe its inflammation, your organs will rest, and your brain will get ready for a new day of challenges. You can pick it all back up in the morning, when you're fresh, and start again.

Bone Broth Tea

When you're overwhelmed or stressed, stop for a moment, take a few deep breaths, and enjoy a soothing cup of broth. The chamomile and lemongrass will help soothe your nervous system.

PREP TIME: 3 min.

COOK TIME: 3 min. and 10 min. wait time

YIELD: 1 serving

1 cup Chicken Bone Broth (page 272) or store-bought

1 chamomile tea bag

1 (1-inch) piece lemongrass or 1 tablespoon freshly squeezed lemon juice

$1/_2$ teaspoon freshly grated peeled fresh ginger

1 handful spinach, coarsely chopped, optional

Pinch of nutmeg, optional

In a small saucepan over high heat, add the bone broth, tea bag, lemongrass, and ginger and bring to a boil. Add the spinach (if using for a more filling broth). Cover, turn off the heat, and steep for about 10 minutes to let the flavors meld. Season with a pinch of nutmeg (if using).

Pot of Gold: Salmon Chowder

Chowder is a great comfort food when you need something soothing. Rather than all the heaviness of New England clam chowder, this one has a lighter and more flavorful broth. When you feel like there's just too much to do and you're always on the run, stop and take a break. Warm up a cup of salmon chowder, put your feet up, and relax.

PREP TIME: 20 min.
COOK TIME: 25 min.
YIELD: 4 to 5 servings

2 strips natural sugar- and nitrate-free turkey bacon, diced, optional

2 tablespoons ghee or pasture-raised butter

1 to 2 leeks (white parts only), thinly sliced (about 1^1/$_2$ cups)

1 celery stalk, diced

1 garlic clove, minced

1 quart (4 cups) Chicken (page 272) or Fish Bone Broth (page 275) or store-bought

1 large waxy potato, peeled and cut into ^{1}/$_2$-inch cubes (see Notes)

1 (14-ounce) can full-fat coconut milk

1 teaspoon fresh or ^{1}/$_2$ teaspoon dried thyme

1 dried bay leaf

1 teaspoon Celtic sea or pink Himalayan salt

^{1}/$_4$ teaspoon freshly ground black pepper

Pinch of ground cayenne pepper

1^1/$_2$ pounds skinless salmon, cut into 1-inch pieces

1 (5-ounce) container or bag baby spinach (about 4 cups loosely packed)

2 tablespoons fresh or 1^1/$_2$ to 2 teaspoons dried dill

In a stockpot over medium heat, cook the bacon (if using) for 7 to 8 minutes or until done. Remove the bacon from the pot and set aside. Add the ghee, leeks, and celery and sauté for 7 to 8 minutes or until softened. Add the garlic and sauté for 1 to 2 minutes. Add the bone broth, increase the heat to medium-high, and bring to a low boil. Add the potatoes, reduce the heat to medium, and simmer for about 10 minutes or until fork tender. Add the coconut milk, thyme, bay leaf, salt, pepper, and cayenne, bring to a simmer, and cook for 3 to 5 minutes. Add the salmon, spinach, dill, and the reserved bacon, reduce the heat to medium-low, cover, and simmer for about 3 to 5 minutes or until the salmon is cooked through. Remove the bay leaf before serving.

Key ingredients for stress reduction: bone broth, garlic, salmon, spinach

NOTE

Waxy potatoes have a thin, papery skin that can be easily scratched off with your fingernail. Red potatoes, new potatoes, Yukon gold potatoes, and fingerling potatoes are all types of waxy potatoes. They have a lower starch content, and given their waxy nature, they hold their shape well as they cook. In contrast, starchy potatoes, such as russets, will fall apart when cooked.

Pot of Gold: Butternut-Apple Soup with Warming Spices

When you're under stress, you need to treat yourself with gentleness and self-soothe as much as possible. Knowing that you're caring for yourself by eating healthful and flavorful meals will make you feel more grounded during hard times. Warming spices, like ginger, turmeric, and cinnamon can feel comforting when your nervous system is overloaded.

PREP TIME: 20 min.
COOK TIME: 30 min.
YIELD: 4 to 6 servings

1 tablespoon ghee or coconut oil

1 leek (white parts only), thinly sliced

1 large apple, peeled and cut into 1-inch cubes

2 carrots, sliced

1 quart (4 cups) Chicken Bone Broth (page 272) or store-bought

1 (1$^1/_2$-pound) butternut squash, cut into 1-inch cubes (about 4 cups; see Notes)

1 (1-inch) piece peeled fresh ginger, grated

1 teaspoon ground turmeric

$^1/_2$ to 1 teaspoon ground cinnamon

1 teaspoon Celtic sea or pink Himalayan salt

$^1/_2$ teaspoon freshly ground black pepper

1 (14-ounce) can full-fat coconut milk

In a large stockpot over medium heat, melt the ghee. Add the leeks, apples, and carrots and sauté for 5 to 7 minutes. Add the bone broth, squash, ginger, turmeric, cinnamon, salt, and pepper. Bring to a simmer, stir, cover, and reduce the heat to low. Simmer for about 30 minutes or until the squash is tender.

Purée with an immersion blender, blender, or food processor until smooth (see Notes). Return the soup to the stockpot (if you used a blender or food processor), stir in the coconut milk, and warm through.

Key ingredients to fight stress: bone broth, carrots, turmeric, ginger, cinnamon

NOTES

Butternut squash is difficult to peel and cube. If you find it peeled and precut, it will save you time in the kitchen.

If you use a blender or food processor, process in batches, covering the top with a clean kitchen towel to avoid getting burned.

Butternut squash soup often has just a touch of sweetness. If you'd like more, you can add stevia, monk fruit, or coconut sugar. For a little punch, add a pinch of cayenne pepper.

You can enhance the flavor of spices by toasting them in a small sauté pan on very low heat. As soon as you smell their fragrance and see a tiny wisp of smoke, immediately remove the pan from heat. Spices burn in seconds after that point.

Pot of Gold: Hearty Beef Vegetable Soup

As a child I remember helping my mom in the kitchen. She would lift me up on a kitchen chair and tie one of her aprons under my arms like a little strapless dress. As she chopped and diced, I filled up small bowls and cups believing I was the perfect helper. I joyfully dumped one vegetable at a time into the pot, thinking my indi-

PREP TIME: 30 min.
COOK TIME: 1 hour
YIELD: 6 servings

vidual additions made the soup even better. Memories like that pull on my heartstrings and make me smile. Sometimes it's the recipes we most closely associate with the people and places we love that bring us the greatest stress relief.

$1^1/_2$ pounds chuck or beef stew meat, cut into $^3/_4$-inch cubes

2 teaspoons Celtic sea or pink Himalayan salt, divided

1 tablespoon extra-virgin olive or avocado oil

1 medium onion, diced

2 medium waxy potatoes, peeled and cut into $^1/_2$-inch dice

3 medium carrots, cut into coins or half-moons

2 celery stalks, diced

1 medium red bell pepper, diced

2 to 3 garlic cloves, minced

1 (14-ounce) can diced tomatoes

1 quart (4 cups) Beef Bone Broth (page 274) or store-bought

1 cup dry red wine or an additional 1 cup bone broth

2 tablespoons Worcestershire sauce

1 dried bay leaf

1 teaspoon dried thyme

1 teaspoon freshly ground black pepper

$^3/_4$ cup frozen green beans (see Note)

$^1/_2$ cup frozen peas

Salt the beef with 1 teaspoon of the salt. In a stockpot or Dutch oven over medium heat, add the oil. When the oil is hot, brown the beef in batches for about 3 to 4 minutes each, flipping the meat so that all sides brown. (Keep the meat in one layer so you don't crowd the pot.) Remove the beef as it finishes and set aside, leaving the oil and brown bits in the pot.

Using the same pot, over medium heat, add the onions, potatoes, carrots, celery, and pepper and sauté 5 to 6 minutes. Add the garlic and sauté for another minute.

Add the beef back to the pot and add the tomatoes, bone broth, wine, Worcestershire sauce, bay leaf, thyme, pepper, and the remaining 1 teaspoon salt. Scrape up any brown bits left in the bottom of the pot using a wooden spoon. Cover and simmer over medium-low heat for 1 hour.

Add the green beans and peas and simmer for another 5 to 10 minutes to warm through. Taste to adjust the seasonings. Remove the bay leaf before serving.

Key ingredients for stress relief: bone broth, beef, potatoes, red wine

NOTE
You can also use fresh green beans. Add them when you add the bone broth.

Pot of Gold: Thai Sweet Potato Soup

I'm a huge fan of Thai food. Thai cuisine is on the top of my favorites list, along with Middle Eastern and Italian cuisines. Many ethnic dishes are too complicated to make at home, but this soup is a breeze, and you'll get to enjoy the fragrant essence of lemongrass. If you haven't cooked with it before, it's a great stress buster

PREP TIME: 15 min.
COOK TIME: 40 min.
YIELD: 5 to 6 servings

and also makes a fabulous tea. Simply chop into pieces (it often comes in bundles of 2 or 3 stalks) and simmer in a pot of water.

3 tablespoons ghee or coconut oil

1 small onion, diced

2 pounds sweet potatoes, peeled and cut into 1-inch cubes (about 5 cups)

2 garlic cloves, minced

1 (1-inch) piece peeled fresh ginger, grated

1 to 2 tablespoons Thai red curry paste (see Notes)

1 quart (4 cups) Chicken Bone Broth (page 272) or store-bought

1 lemongrass stalk, cut into 1-inch pieces

1 (14-ounce) can full-fat coconut milk

1 teaspoon Celtic sea or pink Himalayan salt

$1/2$ teaspoon freshly ground black pepper

$1/4$ cup coarsely chopped fresh cilantro (stems removed), divided

1 small to medium jalapeño, thinly sliced, for garnish, optional

In a stockpot over medium-high heat, add the ghee and onions and sauté for about 4 minutes. Add the sweet potatoes and sauté for another 5 minutes. Add the garlic and ginger and sauté for another 2 minutes. Stir in the curry paste, bone broth, and lemongrass and bring to a simmer. Reduce the heat to medium-low and simmer for about 30 minutes or until the sweet potatoes are soft.

Discard the lemongrass and purée the soup with an immersion blender, blender, or food processor until smooth (see Notes). Return the soup to the stockpot (if you used a blender or food processor), stir in the coconut milk, season with the salt and pepper, and warm through over low heat. Stir in half of the cilantro. Taste to adjust the seasonings, adding more red curry paste by the teaspoon until it reaches your desired spiciness. Garnish with the remaining cilantro and the jalapeño (if using).

Key ingredients to reduce stress: bone broth, sweet potatoes, lemongrass, turmeric, red curry paste (which also contains lemongrass)

NOTES

If you have had red curry paste in the refrigerator for over 6 months, it has likely lost much of its spiciness, so it's time to replace it. When you add the curry to the soup, it's best to add little by little, tasting after it after stirring.

If you use a blender or food processor, process in batches, covering the top with a clean kitchen towel to avoid getting burned.

Baked Egg Cups with Artichokes and Spinach

Try these tasty egg cups for breakfast, brunch, or lunch. They're a cinch to make and a refreshing change from scrambled or fried eggs. They refrigerate well and can be reheated just before serving. They also make a great high-protein snack.

PREP TIME: 5 min.

COOK TIME: 20 min.

YIELD: 12 egg cups, enough for 4 to 6 servings

Avocado or coconut spray oil

2 scallions (white and green parts), thinly sliced

1 packed cup baby spinach, chopped

1 (8-ounce) jar water-packed artichoke hearts, drained and coarsely chopped (about 1 cup)

9 eggs

$1/_2$ teaspoon Celtic sea or pink Himalayan salt

$1/_8$ teaspoon freshly ground black pepper

$1/_4$ teaspoon dried thyme or tarragon

Preheat the oven to 350°F. Spray a 12-cup muffin tin with avocado oil.

Divide the scallions, spinach, and artichokes equally among the muffin cups. (The spinach may pop over the top of the cups until you add the eggs.)

In a medium bowl, whisk together the eggs, salt, pepper, and thyme. Fill the muffin cups three-quarters full with the egg mixture and bake for about 20 minutes or until a toothpick or thin-bladed knife inserted into the center of the egg cup comes out clean.

Key ingredients for stress reduction: eggs, artichokes, spinach

Strawberry-Almond Muffins

Packed with juicy strawberries, these muffins are simply delicious and just as pretty. And they're gluten-free! Enjoy for breakfast or as a midday snack with a cup of tea. They store well in the refrigerator for at least 4 days. Enjoy in moderation.

PREP TIME: 25 min.
COOKING TIME: 25 to 30 min.
YIELD: 12 muffins

Avocado spray oil

1 cup diced fresh strawberries

1 tablespoon maple syrup or honey

2 teaspoons chia seeds

$1/_3$ cup ghee or pasture-raised butter, melted

3 large eggs

$1/_3$ cup honey

$3/_4$ cup coconut or almond milk

$1/_4$ teaspoon pure vanilla or almond extract

1 cup blanched almond flour

$1/_3$ cup coconut flour

$1/_2$ teaspoon baking soda

$1/_4$ teaspoon Celtic sea or pink Himalayan salt

Preheat the oven to 325°F and insert muffin liners into a 12-cup muffin tin. Spray each liner with the avocado oil.

In a small saucepan over low heat, combine the strawberries, maple syrup, and chia seeds. Simmer, stirring occasionally, for 8 to 10 minutes. Remove from the heat and let cool.

In a medium bowl, whisk together the ghee, eggs, honey, nut milk, and vanilla extract and set aside. In another bowl, thoroughly combine the almond flour, coconut flour, baking soda, and salt. Gradually add the wet ingredients to the dry ingredients while stirring. Be sure the mixture is thoroughly combined.

Pour the batter into the muffin cups, filling halfway. Spoon in 1 teaspoon of the strawberry compote, then top with another 1 tablespoon of the batter. Bake for 25 to 30 minutes or until a toothpick or thin-bladed knife inserted into the center of a muffin comes out clean.

Key ingredients for stress reduction: almonds, strawberries

NOTE
These muffins will have a flatter top—not a traditional rounded top like muffins made with wheat flour.

Salmon with Orange-Ginger Marinade

Fatty fishes like salmon are a mega-boost for good health. Studies have shown that the omegas in fatty fish can reduce how mental stress affects cardiovascular health, including heart rate and muscle sympathetic nerve activity, which is part of the "fight or flight" response. Given all that good news, adding salmon to your diet is one of the best things you can do for your health.

PREP TIME: 10 min. and 45 min. wait time
COOK TIME: 5 to 10 min.
YIELD: 4 servings

$^1/_4$ cup extra-virgin olive oil

1 tablespoon toasted sesame oil

$1^1/_2$ tablespoons coconut aminos

2 tablespoons freshly squeezed orange juice

1 teaspoon orange zest

1 tablespoon honey

2 teaspoons grated, peeled fresh ginger

1 garlic clove, grated or finely minced (about 1 teaspoon)

$^1/_2$ small jalapeño, seeded and minced, or $^1/_4$ to $^1/_2$ teaspoon crushed red pepper flakes

4 (4- to 5-ounce) or 1 (16- to 20-ounce) whole salmon fillets

Avocado spray oil

1 to 2 scallions (green parts only), sliced on the diagonal, for garnish

1 tablespoon plus 1 teaspoon toasted sesame seeds, for garnish, optional

4 orange slices, for garnish, optional

In a nonreactive bowl, combine the olive oil, sesame oil, coconut aminos, orange juice, orange zest, honey, ginger, garlic, and jalapeño. Add the salmon and cover tightly. (You can also use a resealable plastic bag for marinating). Refrigerate for 1 hour, occasionally turning the salmon. Do not leave the salmon on the counter to marinate, and do not marinate for longer than 1 hour.

Preheat the broiler to high. Line a baking pan with foil and spray with the avocado oil. Place the salmon on the pan and broil for 7 to 8 minutes. Check for doneness (see Notes)—total broiling time will likely vary between 10 to 15 minutes based on the thickness of the salmon and the temperature of your broiler. If the salmon begins to get too brown, tent with foil.

Garnish with the scallions and the sesame seeds and orange slices (if using).

Key ingredients for stress reduction: salmon, orange juice and zest, ginger

NOTES

Salmon is done when it is opaque and easily flakes. The best and easiest way to check for doneness is with an instant-read thermometer. Fish should cook to 145°F at the thickest part. Another method is to make a small cut with a knife so you can see the center of the fish. It should be opaque throughout and flake easily. As a general guide, cook fish for 5 minutes for every 1 inch of thickness, measuring at the thickest part. Do not overcook the salmon. Fish is delicate and cooks quickly—it will dry out if overcooked. You do not need to turn the salmon when broiling.

Chapter 11

The Face Forward Principle: Great Skin, Great Hair, Great Confidence

Do you remember back in the introduction when I asked you to imagine yourself ten years from now, or twenty, or more? I wanted you to picture that future self, looking amazing and ageless. Not a day older than you look today, with beauty and vitality lighting you up from within.

Well now's the time to revisit that image and goal. Because if you're embracing the breakthrough lifestyle from Part Two (even if you're just beginning!), and problem-solving with these chapters in Part Three, you are, indeed, well on your way to stopping the clock. What's next? Being proactive about your beautiful skin and hair—the outward signs of health and vitality that so many of us struggle to feel confident about. But first, let's take a peek into the past:

Have you ever seen a refrigerator magnet or postcard with the saying, "I wish I was as thin as I was when I thought I was fat?" It strikes a chord with me every time, because I meet women every day who are really focused on what they used to be, instead of what they are now or what they can become.

Here's why: Think back to a thin period in your life. Or think of a picture where you like the way you look. Maybe it was your wedding day? Your kid's fifth birthday? A Fourth of July barbecue? When you look at the photo, chances are there's a long list of facets of your appearance you'd give just about anything to still have right now. That weight, that skin, that hair (give or take the style!).

Now, be real: When that picture was taken, did you feel thin? Did you know you had a glow? Did you appreciate the fullness or the bounce or the color of that hair? Did you feel good enough? Or were you thinking about your flaws, the same as you might be if the picture was taken today?

Believe me when I tell you that I have met more women than I can count who are spending their lives looking back, always a little unhappy and a little unfulfilled because of their appearance. Many of us don't realize it, but when we look in the mirror and think negative thoughts about our hair, skin, posture, or weight, day after day, we slowly chip away at our sense of self-worth. These daily micro-aggressions, silently spewed into the mirror—they add up. They undermine us from the inside out.

Remember that woman we've been talking about who walks through life with je ne sais quoi—who lives with easy grace and confidence? Who looks amazing? Now picture her looking like the version of you in that old picture you love. If you could go back to the day it was taken, would you walk with confidence? Would you feel how graceful and attractive and magnetic you were? Would you recognize that in that moment you had that "it" factor?

Or would you be thinking your arms were a little flabby, or your butt too fat or flat, or your jawline too soft, or that if you could just lose fifteen pounds, you'd be hot? I don't know about you, but I find it hurts to admit that even when I was my trimmest and strongest as a young woman, I rarely had the confidence to realize it.

But I do *now*. I don't play that if-only game with myself anymore. I look in that mirror in the morning and do my damnedest—even on my worst days—to be mindful that the woman I am *right now* is smart, attractive, vibrant, and worthy of love. And then I choose to take good care of her for another day—to eat well and move my body, to prioritize sleep and give myself time for stamina-care. Do I accomplish that perfectly every day? Nobody does. Do I do it *most of the time*? Absolutely.

I can honestly say that this shift in the way I view myself has all but stopped time leaving its mark on my body for more than a decade—and it's a shift you can make, too. I want to make you a confident, beautiful, aging enigma—and the approach that's going to work is what I call the "Face Forward Principle."

Face Forward is what we were really talking about in the first few pages of the book. It's loving and taking care of who you are today, so that in ten or twenty years, you'll still have your "it" factor. I'm not really trying to reinvent the wheel here. I'm just asking you to shift your perspective and ask yourself, *Why not find the beauty today that I'm going to recognize was there some day in the future?* And while you're at it, *Why not choose to live the breakthrough lifestyle that can help me preserve it?* It's a way to see yourself in a whole different light. And I promise you that if you try it, even for a little while, you'll wish you'd been doing it your whole life.

Psychologists tell us that confidence is not an innate, fixed characteristic. You're not born with it. It's an ability you can acquire and improve over time. If you look at someone who has confidence—that woman with je ne sais quoi—you'll see someone who has done the work to improve her sense of self. If you took that away from her, she wouldn't make you sit up and take notice anymore.

Look, aging is inevitable, but that doesn't mean we can't control *how* it happens. We now have scientific evidence to prove we can repair our skin and slow down the process. Let's look at how it's done.

The Thin Line Between Wellness and Beauty

Looking great and feeling great go hand in hand, and there is nothing vain or objectifying about that. If you're doing the work of changing your diet and lifestyle, I have no doubt you're doing it to get healthier. You want to keep up with your kids, your grandkids, your partner, your friends, and the demands of the career and other pursuits that help you feel purposeful, creative, and vibrant. You want to live life to the fullest.

But aren't you also *maybe* . . . hoping you'll look better in the process? I know I sure am. "Beauty" and all that entails—well, it's one of my favorite things to immerse myself in. I like to look nice. That's not a bombshell confession; it's just a little truth most of us share. I like to feel confident and sexy and light on my feet. I like knowing I have a bright smile—and I appreciate bright smiles on everyone else.

I have a friend who has been going through a painful divorce after a decades-long marriage to a man who never treated her with the kindness and respect she deserved. This process has been hard on her, but as I've watched her walk through it, I've been constantly reminded that wellness, confidence, beauty, and happiness—they're all connected. To see this lovely woman, who was once so down she didn't even want to comb her hair, start eating healthfully, walking for thirty minutes at every lunch, hiking with her daughter on the weekend, choosing new clothes and getting her hair styled, *grinning* as she makes plans for what *she* would like for dinner or what movie *she'd* like to watch—well, it kinda makes my heart sing.

Sometimes, the line between wellness and beauty isn't just thin, it's paper thin. I don't want you to ever feel like you need to justify wanting to look good right along with feeling healthy. Do both, and be confident!

Let's Talk about Sunshine

Confused about the sun and the role it plays in your aging, your beauty, your good health?

Join the club. One minute you're hearing dire warnings about it causing skin cancer and premature aging. The next we're talking about how critical sunshine is for healthy sleep, hormone balance, and getting vitamin D—the "sunshine vitamin" that keeps your bones strong and protects you from cancer, depression, diabetes, multiple sclerosis, and heart disease.

So, which is it? Should you be scared sunless or let the sunshine in?

Turns out, like a lot of things, the answer is moderation. The sun is here for us, and we need to learn to use it wisely. A little daily exposure is part of a healthy lifestyle. For example, if you're going out for a ten- to twenty-minute walk in the morning, that's a great time to just head out the door and let the sun touch you with its healing, life-sustaining rays.

But at midday or when your exposure is going to be longer (or for multiple short exposures during the day), that's when sun protection becomes essential. Unfortunately, it's not as simple as just picking up a drugstore sunscreen and hitting the beach. Truth is, most sunscreens contain harmful chemicals—and most offer inadequate protection against UVA rays. And when it comes to those SPF numbers, the FDA has noted that any value greater than 50 is "inherently misleading" because that kind of protection in a chemical concoction doesn't exist.

What do you do if you're going to be hiking in the sun all day or sitting on the beach for hours? A natural, organic sunscreen is a good start. You can find reliable recommendations from the Environmental Working Group's website. Next up, choose physical barriers like hats, long sleeves, and umbrellas. The longer you're going to be out, the more care you should take to keep yourself in that moderate-exposure lane.

Bottom line? Don't be afraid of the sun—just be smart about it. Research shows that sensible sun exposure is perfectly fine for your skin. It's the dose that makes the difference, so just don't overdo it.

A Collagen Revolution and a Bone Broth Connection

Gosh almighty, have you walked into a health-food store lately? If so, you're accosted with collagen *everything* upon arrival. And I'm not even mad about it! The sudden proliferation of collagen in easy-to-eat forms is *important*, because it is so nourishing to your skin, which is nothing less than the largest organ in the human body. Collectively, collagen accounts for about one-third of the protein in your body and about 75% of your skin's "dry" weight (because, of course, the thing we are made *most* of is water).

The word "collagen" originates from the Greek word "kolla," which means "glue." This dates back to the early process of boiling the skin and tendons of animals to make glue. But when we look at collagen in the body we're talking about glue in a different sense. It's the substance that helps skin cells renew and repair themselves. In fact, a systematic review of 805 patients showed oral collagen supplements increase skin elasticity, hydration, and dermal collagen density.

Now, the body makes its own collagen—but like so many of the things that make us beautiful, its production drops off as we age. From the time we're somewhere between eighteen and our late twenties, our bodies lose collagen. Around the age of forty, collagen production declines by about 1 to 1.5% per year.

This is why it's so vital to be deliberate about replenishing those lost stores. I suspect that by now you know how this all ties back to bone broth. It is one of the best natural sources of collagen you can incorporate into your diet—one that will help erase the lines on your face and strengthen your skin and hair. In addition to being high in collagen, bone broth also contains the amino acids glycine and proline—both of which help your body build collagen on its own.

By the way, this is no time to forget about gut health. In fact, your gut and your skin are in constant communication—just like the gut and the brain or the lungs—and there may be no single factor that is more influential in skin wellness than gut health. Drink your bone broth daily. As it repairs and seals your gut, hydrates your cells, sates your body with minerals, and doses you with collagen, it serves as the ultimate food in making sure your Face Forward efforts are a success.

Foods You Can Use

In addition to bone broth, there are many foods that benefit your skin while also helping to keep you thin! That's why when people change their diet and lose weight, they also look younger. Nutrition is required for all biological processes of skin—which means what you eat can help or it can hurt. The trouble foods are the ones we keep coming back to as gut-wreckers: sugar, gluten, grains, and dairy are the big offenders. But we've talked enough about those. Let's focus on the foods that can help you get your skin plump and glowing. The easiest way to remember them is to think of them as your ACEs:

Vitamin A: Excellent sources include broccoli, cantaloupe, carrots, collard greens, mangoes, red peppers, spinach, sweet potatoes, tomatoes, and watermelon.

Vitamin C: Excellent sources include asparagus, bananas, blueberries, broccoli, cabbage, cantaloupe, cauliflower, collard greens, mangoes, mustard greens, peaches, pineapple, romaine lettuce, spinach, sweet potatoes, Swiss chard, tomato juice, and watermelon. Note that some foods are on both of these lists—don't you love it when you find a dietary twofer?

Vitamin E: Almonds, hazelnuts, peanuts, and sunflower seeds.

Now here's an important thing to remember about your anti-aging ACE vitamins: They are fat soluble. This means these vitamins require small amounts of dietary fat to help the body absorb, transport, and utilize them. That's why drizzling the vegetables on this list with a heart-healthy oil like olive or avocado can go a long way! Or with fruits and berries, combine them with some nuts—like a handful of blueberries with a handful of almonds. It's a vitamin C and E power-combo snack.

Supplements for Suppleness

It's a wonderful and weird compliment to be told you have great skin—especially if the person giving that compliment assumes you come by it because of great genes. Believe me: you can inherit the potential for an exquisite epidermis from Mom and Dad, but if you don't nurture and protect it, sooner or later you'll still dry out, get dull, wrinkle, and develop any number of skin conditions, from acne to rosacea and beyond. Good skin takes work! It starts with nourishing a healthy gut and eating healthy foods, but I'm happy to tell you there is one shortcut in this area of wellness and beauty. With a healthy diet in place, you can augment it as needed with supplements that build glowing skin from the inside out.

The fact is, even though some topically applied products can penetrate the surface layers of your skin and provide benefits, there's little to no evidence that they can reach the deepest layers—the ones responsible for strength and elasticity.

With this in mind, over the past decade I've banished skin-damaging grains and sugars from my diet and loaded up on skin-renewing foods like bone broth, avocados, coconut oil, blueberries, and leafy greens. The result? I look younger than I did ten years ago. That's what Face Forward is all about!

Now the easy part: besides eating healthy foods, I augment my diet with a handful of supplements that help heal, smooth, and beautify—and I generally recommend my patients do the same. You see, while I believe food should always be your primary source of nutrients, supplements are often also necessary. Especially if you're still working on getting your gut healthy. Once you've accomplished that, your body will be much more efficient at extracting and absorbing the food nutrients you need to keep your glow.

Here are the ones I recommend (and I also recommend letting your doctor know about any supplements you take regularly to ensure none of them will impact your prescription meds):

Collagen

Here it is, again! It's no contest—collagen easily earns the number one spot on my list. It's your skin's "support system," and when it breaks down as you age, your skin starts to sag and wrinkle. In fact, numerous studies have shown that collagen powder (aka hydrolyzed collagen) is readily absorbed by the body and efficiently transported to the deepest layers of your skin where it works its magic. In addition to drinking bone broth, which supplies you with the building blocks of collagen, blast your wrinkles with collagen-powder shakes and smoothies.

How to Buy Collagen

Oral collagen supplements are available in the form of pills and powders. But so many choices can lead to a lot of confusion, so let's break this down. The body can't absorb collagen in its whole form, so the protein needs to be broken down during the digestive process before it absorbs into your bloodstream. What that means for a shopper is that choosing a collagen that is bioavailable (able to be utilized by your body) needs to be a priority. The key word here is "hydrolyzed." That means the collagen is broken down into smaller components called "peptides" that can be more easily absorbed by your digestive tract.

So, when you read labels on collagen products, look for the words "hydrolyzed" and/or "peptides" on the packaging. And if you see collagen sold with vitamin C, that's a plus. Vitamin C is critical for the formation of collagen, so it's great to have it already in the mix.

You may be wondering if sipping on bone broth is enough, or if you also should take supplemental collagen. If you enjoy bone broth and are drinking two cups a day, you're getting enough collagen to significantly nourish your skin and soothe inflammation.

However, if you're not a regular bone broth drinker or if you are dealing with a lot of inflammation or skin issues, you can add a powdered supplement for an extra dose without worry of overdoing it. There are no known health issues linked to the consumption of too much collagen.

Probiotics and Prebiotics

We talked about food forms of these in chapters 7 and 8, but you can also get them in supplement form. These two work hand in hand. Probiotics are beneficial to gut microbes, while prebiotics provide the healthy fiber that helps your microbes thrive. And both are powerful gut healers, which means they may help alleviate skin conditions that cause redness and irritation.

Vitamin C

Your body cannot synthesize new collagen without vitamin C. Period. This is one of the reasons why vitamin C is highly concentrated in the skin. That's where it helps produce fibroblasts—cells necessary for collagen production as well as wound healing. Vitamin C also works as an antioxidant to protect your skin from UV damage—*and* it works to neutralize free radicals caused by toxins. In a world filled with chemicals and pollution, the work vitamin C does is invaluable.

One more thing about this super nutrient: There's evidence suggesting vitamin C plays a role in the production of lipids in the outer layer of your skin. These lipids prevent water loss to keep your skin moist and supple.

Like so many nutrients, vitamin C doesn't work in a bubble. It relies on other enzymes and nutrients, such as vitamin E, carotenoids, and glutathione. That's why I recommend taking vitamin C as part of an antioxidant complex or multivitamin—and also eating a rainbow of colorful fruits and vegetables.

Vitamin E

Vitamin E supports healthy skin due to its antioxidant activity. However, it also works at the immune level to benefit your skin. For example, one study found that almost 50% of participants with atopic dermatitis experienced a significant improvement in their condition with vitamin E supplementation. And 14% of participants experienced complete remission. Less than 1% of participants given a placebo experienced significant improvement or remission.

It is estimated that over 90% of Americans are deficient in vitamin E, partly because the standard American diet is extremely nutrient deficient, and partly because vitamin E is fat-soluble. That means it must be consumed with fat in order for your body to absorb it. No matter your diet, though, it can be difficult to get adequate amounts of vitamin E solely from your food. That's why this is another excellent component to look for in an antioxidant complex or multivitamin.

Vitamin D

If we get technical about it, vitamin D is actually not a vitamin at all, but rather a hormone. It is produced by the skin as a result of unprotected sun exposure. Thus, it can be tricky to get enough—especially since it's not highly concentrated in food.

Research has linked vitamin D deficiencies to several skin conditions, so I recommend taking a supplement that combines vitamin D and vitamin K, as well as occasionally having your levels tested to be sure you're getting enough.

Zinc

This trace mineral is found in relatively high concentrations in your skin compared to other tissues in your body. Zinc is an amazing skin strengthener because it's involved in protein synthesis, DNA synthesis, collagen production, cell division, and even your immune response. Plus, it has antioxidant properties to help protect your skin cells from damage.

Magnesium

Magnesium helps the body relax and ease stress—and stress is a big factor when it comes to healthy skin (especially in the case of stress-induced acne).

CoQ10

CoQ10 is a potent antioxidant found in some foods, and it's also produced by your body. However, production naturally decreases as you age. A handful of studies has shown that supplemental CoQ10 may offer some pretty (pun intended) nice benefits for your skin. For example, one study found that supplementing with CoQ10 helped improve visual signs of aging, such as wrinkles, fine lines, and rough skin.

Detox-and-Hydrate Happy Hour

Here's a simple nutrition, skin care, and stamina-care hack you can indulge in every day: infusion cocktails. Truth is, if you want beautiful, healthy skin, you've got to drink your water. Skin-care experts talk a lot about moisturizing, but you can only nourish and plump your skin so much from the outside. Hydration is what we need to aim for, and it's strictly an inside job—accomplished when you drink plenty of fluids and eat your fruits and veggies.

It's amazing how many women I meet who pull a face at the idea of drinking plain old ho-hum water. But I get it—we want *more*. A little joy with our H_2O. Luckily, you can improve on the flavor of water in ways that are magic for your skin—just by throwing some sliced or diced fruits and vegetables into the glass and letting them soak. These water "cocktails" are delish if you drink right after making them, but to get the most from your effort, consider prepping them before bed and letting them steep in the fridge overnight. There is something about a cool pitcher of cucumber water that says "first class," don't you think? Like it's caviar or champagne or something equally fancy, rather than just, well, cucumbers and water.

Some of my other favorite alcohol-free hydration cocktails include:

- Melon-cucumber mix: Fresh and refreshing—at least as good as an Arnold Palmer on a hot day.
- Lime and crushed mint: A mojito without the rum. Lime is a natural diuretic that helps you detox, and mint soothes the body from the inside out, calming your digestive system and supporting good skin health.
- Coconut-pineapple infusion: Soak pineapple chunks in coconut water for a piña colada–esque experience at any time of the day or night.
- And my number one standby for morning hydration: zippy, cleansing, invigorating lemon water. My favorite now and forever.

Now, we all know that the other breakthrough lifestyle factors are critical to good skin. The fact is, when we talk about "beauty rest," we're not kidding. Nobody wants to look tired—even when they are. I frequently remind my patients of this in terms even a child can understand: Regular, quality sleep makes you a Sleeping Beauty. But skimping? It'll make you an Eeyore in a hurry.

And then there's exercise—the great problem-solving, beautifying, health-enhancing magic trick we all need to make time for as often as we can. We tend to only focus on exercise to lose weight and protect our heart health. But exercise improves blood circulation—and anything that improves circulation is going to keep your skin healthy and vibrant. And sweating rids the body of harmful toxins that can damage your skin. You don't have to run a marathon. You don't have to climb a mountain. Find your body vibe and engage in a physical activity you love, and all the anti-aging magic of exercise will be yours.

Collagen-Powered Bone Broth

Broth, collagen peptides, and avocado support your skin with loads of collagen and healthful fats to help keep you soft, supple, and smooth.

PREP TIME: 5 min.

COOK TIME: 3 min. and 10 min. wait time

YIELD: 1 serving

1 cup Chicken Bone Broth (page 272) or store-bought, plus more as needed

1 scoop collagen peptides

Handful of watercress or spinach, coarsely chopped

$\frac{1}{4}$ avocado, diced small

1 teaspoon freshly squeezed lemon or lime juice

Pinch of Celtic sea or pink Himalayan salt

Pinch of freshly ground black pepper

1 to 2 tablespoons chopped fresh cilantro (stems removed)

In a small saucepan over high heat, add the bone broth and collagen peptides and bring to a boil. Add the watercress, avocado, and lemon juice. Cover the pot, turn off the heat, and steep for about 10 minutes to let the flavors meld. Season with the salt and pepper and top with cilantro.

NOTE

If you want a creamy texture, you can whiz the soup in a blender, but you may need to reheat it.

Arugula Salad with Pomegranate Vinaigrette

I love the peppery spice of fresh arugula. It's a great starting point for many salads. In this recipe, I use pomegranate juice and arils because of their tart and sweet flavor profile. This combo is the perfect counterpoint to the spiciness of the arugula.

PREP TIME: 10 min.

YIELD: 4 servings

$^1/_2$ cup pomegranate juice

$^1/_2$ small shallot, minced (about 1$^1/_2$ to 2 tablespoons)

1 to 2 garlic cloves, smashed

1 (5-ounce) container baby arugula

1 apple, sliced or diced

1 medium beet, grated or spiralized, then coarsely chopped

1 avocado, sliced or diced

$^1/_3$ English cucumber, cut into half moons

4 tablespoons walnuts or pistachios, toasted and very coarsely chopped, divided

$^1/_2$ cup extra-virgin olive oil

2 teaspoons balsamic vinegar

2 to 3 teaspoons honey or maple syrup

1 teaspoon Dijon mustard

Pinch of Celtic sea or pink Himalayan salt

2 tablespoons pomegranate arils, optional

4 to 6 ounces sheep's or goat's milk feta or shaved Manchego cheese, optional

In a small saucepan over low heat, add the pomegranate juice, shallots, and garlic and gently simmer for 10 to 15 minutes or until it is reduced by half. Keep the heat low and do not boil. Remove from the heat and set aside to cool for about 30 minutes.

Meanwhile, in a large bowl, toss together the arugula, apple, beet, avocado, cucumber, and 2 tablespoons of the walnuts.

When the pomegranate reduction is cool, discard the garlic and add the olive oil, vinegar, honey, mustard, and salt and whisk together.

Top the salad with the remaining 2 tablespoons walnuts, the arils, and cheese (if using). Dress the salad or serve the dressing on the side.

Key ingredients for anti-aging: pomegranate, pistachios, walnuts

Pot of Gold: Creamy Avocado Soup with Mango Salsa

Your skin needs hydration and collagen to stay soft and supple. With collagen from the bone broth and healthy oil from the avocados, this soup gives your body what it needs to keep your skin dewy and glowing. The sweet and spicy mango salsa adds a whole new depth of flavor to the avocado soup. If you have leftover

PREP TIME: 20 min.
COOK TIME: 20 min.
YIELD: 4 to 5 servings

mango salsa, enjoy it as a delicious accompaniment to fish or tacos, or toss several tablespoons into a garden salad for a pop of sweet and spicy deliciousness. In lieu of the salsa, there are several other soup toppings in the Notes that you might enjoy.

FOR THE SOUP:

- 2 tablespoons avocado oil
- 1 small onion, diced (about $^1/_2$ cup)
- 1 garlic clove, minced
- 1 quart (4 cups) Chicken Bone Broth (page 272) or store-bought
- 2 ripe avocados, cut into chunks
- 1 cup full-fat coconut milk (from a can)
- $^1/_4$ cup freshly squeezed lime juice (from about 2 limes)
- $^1/_2$ cup fresh cilantro, stems removed
- $^1/_2$ to 1 teaspoon ground coriander
- 1 teaspoon Celtic sea or pink Himalayan salt
- $^1/_2$ teaspoon freshly black pepper

FOR THE MANGO SALSA:

- 2 ripe mangoes, cut into $^1/_4$-inch dice
- $^1/_2$ red bell pepper, cut into $^1/_4$-inch dice
- $^1/_4$ small red onion, cut into $^1/_4$-inch dice (about $^1/_4$ cup)
- $^1/_2$ small jalapeño, seeded and finely minced (about 2 tablespoons)
- 2 tablespoons freshly squeezed lime juice (from about 1 lime)
- 2 tablespoons coarsely chopped fresh cilantro (stems removed)
- $^1/_4$ to $^1/_2$ teaspoon Celtic sea or pink Himalayan salt

Make the soup: In a stockpot over medium heat, add the avocado oil and onions and sauté for 7 to 8 minutes or until soft. Add the garlic and sauté for another 1 to 2 minutes.

Add the broth, avocados, coconut milk, lime juice, cilantro, coriander, salt, and pepper and simmer for 15 to 20 minutes. Purée with an immersion blender, food processor, or blender (see Note). Serve with the mango salsa.

Make the salsa: In a medium bowl, add the mangoes, bell pepper, onion, jalapeño, lime juice, cilantro, and salt. Toss together and refrigerate so flavors can meld while the soup cooks.

Key ingredients for anti-aging: bone broth, avocados, avocado oil, jalapeño, red bell pepper

---

NOTES

If you decide to skip the mango salsa, any number of ingredients make excellent toppings for this soup. A few of my favorites are onions or scallions, chopped cilantro, salsa fresca, chopped tomatoes, a drizzle of olive oil, toasted pepitas, or hot sauce.

If you use a blender or food processor, process in batches, covering the top with a clean kitchen towel to avoid getting burned.

If you enjoy hot and smoky flavors, consider adding smoked paprika, ground chipotle powder, or chipotle in adobo to the soup. If you use the latter, add before blending. Start with half of a chipotle pepper and 1 to 2 teaspoons of the adobo sauce. You can always add more.

If you want to thin the soup, add a little more bone broth. To make the soup even creamier, add more coconut milk.

Pot of Gold: Bloody Mary Gazpacho

Do you enjoy an occasional bloody or virgin Mary with brunch? Here it is as a chilled soup. I say cheers to that! Gazpacho is loaded with good-for-you ingredients to keep you strong and youthful. Enjoy a cup or bowl on a sizzling summer day, kick back, and relax. You deserve to take some time for yourself. I know what you're thinking, so I thought I should answer before you ask: yes, you can add a shot of vodka to your gazpacho, just don't overdo it. Gazpacho is also very satiating when you're feeling hungry between meals.

PREP TIME: 15 min.
YIELD: 4 to 6 servings

- 2 cups Beef (page 274) or Chicken Bone Broth (page 272) or store-bought, divided
- 4 medium ripe tomatoes, quartered (about 1 pound), or 1 (14-ounce) can diced tomatoes
- 2 tablespoons extra-virgin olive oil
- 1 garlic clove, minced
- 2 tablespoons freshly squeezed lemon or lime juice
- 2 to 3 teaspoons prepared horseradish (see Notes)
- 1 to 2 teaspoons Worcestershire sauce (see Notes)
- 1 to 2 teaspoons Tabasco sauce or other hot sauce (see Notes)

- 1 teaspoon Celtic sea or pink Himalayan salt
- 1 teaspoon freshly ground black pepper
- 1 English cucumber, cut into 1- to 2-inch chunks
- 1 red bell pepper, cut into 1- to 2-inch chunks
- 3 celery stalks, cut into 1-inch pieces
- $1/4$ small red onion, very coarsely chopped
- $1/4$ to $1/2$ jalapeño, seeded and coarsely chopped, optional
- 2 tablespoons coarsely chopped fresh cilantro or flat-leaf parsley (stems removed), optional

In a blender or food processor, combine 1 cup of the bone broth, the tomatoes, olive oil, garlic, lemon juice, horseradish, Worcestershire sauce, Tabasco, salt, and pepper. Blend until smooth. Pour into a large bowl and set aside.

In the same blender or food processor, add the remaining 1 cup bone broth, the cucumber, bell pepper, celery, onion, jalapeño, and the cilantro (if using). Pulse until chunky (the texture should be similar to salsa fresca). Add to the tomato mixture, stir to combine, and taste to adjust the seasonings as desired.

Key ingredients for anti-aging: bone broth, tomatoes, red bell pepper, olive oil, jalapeños

NOTES

I included a range of measurements for the horseradish, Worcestershire sauce, Tabasco, and jalapeño because everyone likes a different level of umami (from the Worcestershire) or heat. Start small; you can always add more.

There are many fabulous garnishes for gazpacho that you might like: cubed avocado, celery, red bell pepper, cucumbers, shrimp, a drizzle of olive oil, cilantro, or parsley. If you like a smoky flavor, you can add a dash of smoked paprika.

Pot of Gold: Broccoli "Cheese" Soup

If you haven't used nutritional yeast in the past, you'll be delighted to discover that it tastes like cheese. Nutritional yeast, also called "nooch," is an inactive version of the same yeast used for baking bread and brewing beer, but since it's not "active," you can't use it for either. It comes in flakes, granules, or powder, and it's usually found in the spice or baking section at the su-permarket. At a more natural grocery store, you'll also find it in bulk. Nutritional yeast is low in sodium and calories, and it's fat-free, sugar-free, and gluten-free. It's used often in vegan cooking as a stand-in for cheese. I think you're going to be pleasantly surprised!

PREP TIME: 15 min. and 4 hrs. wait time

COOK TIME: 30 min.

YIELD: 6 to 7 servings

1 cup raw cashews

2 tablespoons avocado oil or ghee

1 small onion, diced

2 celery stalks, diced

2 carrots, diced

1 to 2 garlic cloves, minced

1 quart (4 cups) Chicken Bone Broth (page 272) or store-bought

1 medium Yukon gold potato, peeled and diced into 1-inch cubes

$^3/_4$ pound broccoli, cut into small florets (about 4 cups)

1 cup full-fat coconut milk (from a can)

$^1/_2$ cup nutritional yeast

1 teaspoon ground turmeric

1 teaspoon Celtic sea or pink Himalayan salt

$^1/_2$ teaspoon freshly ground black pepper

In a small bowl, cover the cashews with cool water and soak for 4 hours. Rinse and drain and set aside.

In a large stockpot over medium-high heat, add the avocado oil, onions, celery, and carrots and sauté for 7 to 8 minutes. Add the garlic and sauté for another minute. Add the bone broth, increase the heat to high, and bring to a low boil. Add the po-tato and broccoli, reduce the heat to medium, and simmer for about 15 minutes or until the potato is soft. Stir in the reserved cashews, the coconut milk, nutritional yeast, turmeric, salt, and pepper and simmer for 7 to 8 minutes. Purée with an im-mersion blender, blender, or food processor (see Notes).

Key ingredients for anti-aging: bone broth, broccoli

NOTES

If you use a blender or food processor, process in batches, covering the top with a clean kitchen towel to avoid getting burned.

This is a very thick and creamy soup. You may want to add more bone broth if you like your soup a bit thinner.

Salmon Tacos with Cabbage Slaw and Creamy Cilantro Dressing

These salmon tacos are sure to delight the entire family, and the cabbage slaw is so delicious you'll probably find yourself making it as a side dish with other meals. Lime juice adds a refreshing citrus note that compliments the creamy dressing. Don't skip the salsa fresca or diced tomatoes to top off the tacos. Tomatoes add another anti-aging component to the meal,

PREP TIME: 15 min.

COOK TIME: 10 min.

YIELD: 8 tacos, enough for 4 servings

as well as a bright splash of color and flavor. If you're not a fan of grain-free taco shells or just prefer a simpler meal, this is fantastic as a salmon-and-salad feast.

FOR THE CABBAGE SALAD:

$1/_2$ cup extra-virgin olive oil

1 avocado

1 bunch fresh cilantro, stems removed, very coarsely chopped

1 garlic clove

3 tablespoons freshly squeezed lime juice (from about $1^1/_2$ limes)

$1/_2$ teaspoon ground coriander

$1/_2$ teaspoon Celtic sea or pink Himalayan salt

3 cups green or napa cabbage, very thinly sliced

1 small red bell pepper, cut into $1/_4$-inch dice

FOR THE TACOS:

Avocado spray oil

1 (1-pound) salmon fillet

$1/_2$ teaspoon Celtic sea or pink Himalayan salt

$1/_4$ teaspoon freshly ground black pepper

8 grain-free taco shells

Diced tomatoes or salsa fresca, for garnish, optional

Sliced jalapeño, for garnish, optional

Make the cabbage salad: In a blender or food processor, combine the olive oil, avocado, cilantro, garlic, lime juice, coriander, and salt. Purée for 2 to 3 minutes or until combined.

In a medium bowl, add the cabbage and bell pepper. Toss with the dressing and refrigerate so the flavors can meld.

Make the tacos: Preheat the broiler to high and generously spray a baking pan with the avocado oil.

Place the salmon on the baking pan and season with the salt and pepper. Broil for about 5 minutes. Check for doneness (see Notes). The total baking time will range from 5 to 8 minutes depending on the thickness of the fillet.

Warm or toast the taco shells in the oven at 400°F or in a dry sauté pan over medium-high heat for 2-3 minutes. Flake the salmon and divide among the tacos. Top with the cabbage slaw. Garnish with the tomatoes and jalapeño (if using).

Key ingredients for anti-aging: salmon, avocados, avocado oil, tomatoes, jalapeño

NOTES

Salmon is done when it is opaque and easily flakes. The best and easiest way to check for doneness is with an instant-read thermometer. Fish should cook to 145°F at the thickest part. Another method is to make a small cut with a knife so you can see the center of the fish. It should be opaque throughout and flake easily. As a general guide, cook fish for 5 minutes for every 1 inch of thickness, measuring at the thickest part. Do not overcook the salmon. Fish is delicate and cooks quickly—it will dry out if overcooked. You do not need to turn the salmon when broiling.

If you have extra slaw, enjoy it as a side dish with seafood or chicken. You could even double the recipe to make sure you have leftovers for other meals. It gets better after being in the refrigerator overnight. You can also make the cilantro dressing to use in salads, with crudités, or to serve with almost any fish or chicken.

Ahi Tuna with Tahini-Lime Sauce

I love to marinate tuna—it easily absorbs the aromatics from this marinade, which adds so much oomph. This simple marinade is a medley of Asian seasonings that are a balance of umami, sour, salty, and spice. The tahini sauce is completely optional but delicious. (It's also a fabulous salad dressing.) Before running off to the supermarket, read the Notes to learn more about ahi tuna, as well as how to make a sesame crust.

PREP TIME: 15 min. and 2 hrs. wait time

COOK TIME: 3 min.

YIELD: 4 servings

FOR THE TAHINI-LIME SAUCE:

$1/_3$ cup tahini, well-stirred (see Notes)

$1/_4$ cup freshly squeezed lime juice (from about 2 limes)

1 tablespoon coconut aminos

2 teaspoons honey

2 to 3 dashes of hot sauce or $1/_4$ teaspoon crushed red pepper flakes, plus more as needed

Pinch of Celtic sea or pink Himalayan salt

FOR THE MARINADE AND TUNA:

$2/_3$ cup plus 1 tablespoon avocado oil, divided, plus more as needed

2 tablespoons toasted sesame oil

3 to 4 tablespoons coconut aminos

2 tablespoons freshly squeezed lime juice (from about 1 lime)

1 tablespoon grated peeled fresh ginger

3 to 4 garlic cloves, minced

2 dashes of hot sauce

4 (4- to 6-ounce) sushi-grade ahi tuna steaks (see Notes)

Make the tahini-lime sauce: In a small bowl or blender, add the tahini, lime juice, coconut aminos, honey, hot sauce, and salt and mix. Add water, 1 tablespoon at a time, until you get the consistency you want (you may end up using 3 to 6 tablespoons; see Notes). Refrigerate until ready to use.

Make the tuna: In a nonreactive bowl, whisk together the $2/_3$ cup avocado oil, the sesame oil, coconut aminos, lime juice, ginger, garlic, and hot sauce. Add the tuna to the marinade, cover, and refrigerate for 2 hours. (You can also use a resealable plastic bag for marinating.)

Place a large sauté pan over medium-high to high heat (using a cast-iron pan will give you the best results). When hot, add the remaining 1 tablespoon avocado oil and heat until shimmering. Add the tuna and sear for 30 to 90 seconds, forming a slight crust; flip and sear the other side. The inside should remain pink. You may want to cook in two batches to avoid crowding. If so, you may need to use more oil. Again, be sure it's very hot.

Serve with the tahini-lime sauce on the side.

Key ingredients for anti-aging: bone broth, tuna, ginger, hot sauce

---

NOTES

Sushi-grade ahi tuna is yellowfin tuna that has been flash-frozen as soon as it is caught, killing any bacteria and parasites. *Saku* tuna is another name for sushi-grade ahi. It is cut into a boneless, skinless block, vacuum sealed, and frozen. This is often used in restaurants because it results in uniform rectangular slices.

If you'd like to make a sesame crust for the tuna, spread $1/4$ cup or more of black or white sesame seeds (or a mixture of both) on a plate. When removing the tuna from the marinade, let the excess liquid drip off, and then place the fish on top of the sesame seeds. Coat one side, pressing to embed the seeds. Flip to coat the second side, firmly pressing the seeds into the fish.

If your tuna is not sushi grade, you should fully cook it over medium heat to an internal temperature of 145°F. Make sure to skip the sesame crust because it will burn, and brush the tuna with extra avocado oil to keep it moist. Depending on the thickness of your fillet, it could take 4 to 5 minutes per side.

Because tahini is made from ground sesame seeds, the sesame oil in it tends to separate, making it difficult to recombine. If it's totally separated, you may need to use a blender. This sauce also makes a delicious salad dressing, but you might want to thin it even more.

Chocolate Pudding with Crunchy Grain-Free Granola

This pudding is packed with healthy ingredients . . . and it's a decadent, creamy, chocolatey dessert. You can also enjoy the pudding or the granola on their own. Ahhhh, life is so good! Don't be daunted by the list of ingredients in the granola. They're just nuts and seeds, and you can mix and match as you choose. You'll also have extra granola to enjoy for breakfasts or snacks (see Notes). You can also buy grain-free granola if you'd prefer not to make it.

PREP TIME: 10 min. for the pudding and 10 min. for the granola

COOK TIME: 25 minutes for the granola

YIELD: 4 to 6 servings pudding, 5 to 5 $1/2$ cups granola

FOR THE GRAIN-FREE GRANOLA:

$1/4$ cup coconut oil, melted

$1/4$ cup maple syrup, warmed

1 teaspoon pure vanilla or almond extract

1 cup raw sunflower seeds

1 cup unsweetened coconut flakes

1 cup raw pepitas

2 cups raw unsalted nuts, such as cashews, pecans, walnuts, sliced or slivered almonds, or any combination you prefer

2 tablespoons chia seeds

2 tablespoons ground flax meal

$1/2$ teaspoon Celtic sea or pink Himalayan salt

$1^1/2$ teaspoons ground cinnamon, optional

FOR THE PUDDING:

$1/4$ cup stevia- or monk-fruit-sweetened chocolate chips, melted (see Notes)

2 large avocados

$1/4$ cup cacao or natural cocoa powder

2 tablespoons cashew, almond, or sesame-seed butter

$1/2$ cup coconut cream

Make the granola: Place an oven rack in the center of the oven and preheat it to 300°F. Line a sheet pan with parchment paper or a silicone mat. Depending on the size of your sheet pan, you may need two.

In a large bowl, combine the coconut oil, maple syrup, and vanilla. Add the sunflower seeds, coconut flakes, pepitas, nuts, chia seeds, flax meal, salt, and cinnamon (if using). Stir well to fully combine. Spread the mixture out evenly on the baking sheet(s).

Bake for 15 minutes, remove from the oven, and stir. Bake for another 10 minutes, carefully watching to make sure it doesn't burn. The coconut should brown at the edges and the nuts should be golden. Depending on your oven and how many pans you use, you may need to continue baking in 3- to 5-minute intervals. Nuts burn very easily so continue to watch closely.

Let the granola cool on the pan and then store it in a sealed container in the freezer for freshness.

Make the pudding: In a food processor, add the chocolate, avocado, cacao, cashew butter, and coconut cream. Purée until smooth and creamy. Pour the pudding into individual serving dishes. Sprinkle with 3 tablespoons of the grain-free granola and refrigerate to set before serving.

Key ingredients for anti-aging: avocados, cocoa, dark chocolate, sunflower seeds, pepitas, nuts, chia seeds, flaxseed

NOTES
Because this granola recipe makes 5 to 5 $\frac{1}{2}$ cups, you will have about 4 to 4 $\frac{1}{2}$ cups left over to enjoy with your favorite nut milk or coconut yogurt. It's also great sprinkled on a salad for added crunch. You can cut the recipe in half for equally reliable results, but you might need the full amount of maple syrup and coconut oil to coat the nuts and seeds.

To melt the chocolate chips, place them in a microwave-safe bowl and cook in 5-second intervals. You're only melting $\frac{1}{4}$ cup, so it won't take more than a few seconds.

Lemon Cheesecake Bars with Berry Topping

We all need a treat sometimes, and this refreshing lemony cheesecake with no dairy fills the bill—all the while giving you an extra dose of skin-nourishing ingredients. Yes, you heard me right: no dairy in these bars, and they are absolutely divine. Raw cashews stand in for cream cheese, and they create the smooth, luscious texture of a traditional cheesecake. You can even share this one with your vegan friends! Try it with the berry topping to make it a special-occasion treat.

PREP TIME: 20 min. plus 1 hr. wait time

CHILL TIME: 3-plus hrs.

YIELD: 16 servings

FOR THE CHEESECAKE:

$1^1/_2$ cups raw unsalted cashews

Avocado spray oil

$^3/_4$ cup unsweetened full-fat coconut milk (from a can)

$^1/_3$ cup coconut oil, melted

$^1/_3$ cup freshly squeezed lemon juice (from about $2^1/_2$ lemons)

2 teaspoons finely grated fresh lemon zest

$1^1/_2$ teaspoons pure vanilla extract

$^1/_3$ cup coconut sugar or honey

Pinch of Celtic sea or pink Himalayan salt

FOR THE BERRY TOPPING:

2 cups berries, such as blueberries, blackberries, raspberries, strawberries, or any combination you prefer

2 teaspoons coconut sugar

$^1/_2$ teaspoon pure vanilla extract

Fresh peppermint leaves, for garnish

Make the cheesecake: In a medium saucepan over high heat, bring 4 cups of water to a boil. Remove from the heat, add the cashews, cover, and let stand for 1 hour. (Or you can soak the cashews in 4 cups of water and refrigerate overnight.) Spray an 8 × 8-inch baking pan or casserole dish with the avocado oil. Cut two pieces of parchment paper long enough to hang over the edges of the pan and line the pan by laying them one across the other. (That little bit of extra length on each side will give you a handy sling for lifting the bars out so you can serve perfect squares every time.)

Drain and rinse the cashews in cold water. In a food processor, add the cashews, coconut milk, coconut oil, lemon juice, lemon zest, vanilla, coconut sugar, and salt and purée for about 5 minutes or until creamy and pourable.

Pour the mixture into the prepared pan. Cover and chill in the refrigerator for 2 hours.

Make the berry topping: In a small saucepan over medium-low heat, combine the berries and coconut sugar. Simmer for 8 to 10 minutes or until the mixture is saucy but the fruit still retains some of its shape. Remove from the heat and add the vanilla. Refrigerate for about 1 hour or freeze for 20 minutes before using.

Remove the cheesecake from the refrigerator and score into 16 squares. (The cheesecake will still be soft, but scoring will make it easier to cut after freezing.) Freeze for 30 to 60 minutes to achieve your preferred firmness.

Use the parchment sling to remove the cheesecake from the baking pan. Cut through the lines you scored earlier to make 16 individual bars. Serve with berry topping (if using) and the peppermint leaves.

Key ingredients for healthy skin and hair: cashews, lemon, berries

---

NOTES

Variations on this one include a sprinkling of any fresh berries, a dollop of coconut whipped cream, or a sprig of mint, fresh thyme, or rosemary. Yummy every way you make it!

Appendix: Dr. Kellyann's Bone Broth Recipes from Scratch

If you're like me (with my busy schedule), sometimes you have time to make bone broth at home, and sometimes you've got to get it at the market or order it in. And of course, sometimes it takes a tea kettle and a packet of bone broth powder from a purse or desk drawer to save the day!

The best thing about making broth at home (besides that fresh taste) is that you can make enough to last awhile. I typically fill mason jars with enough from each batch to last 3 to 4 days, mix some into my favorite soup recipes, and freeze a few portions for the following week. That's a lot of return on investment for my afternoon in the kitchen.

One extra tip from my stockpot to yours: To amp up the flavor of your broth, add any of these tasty, metabolism-boosting spices to the pot: 2 teaspoons sliced peeled ginger, a handful of parsley or cilantro, 1 teaspoon ground turmeric, a pinch of ground cayenne pepper, or 1 to 2 teaspoons ground cumin.

Chicken Bone Broth

PREP TIME: 15 min.

COOK TIME: 6 to 8 hrs.

YIELD: Varies depending on size of pot; these ingredients are sufficient for 1 gallon of broth

3-plus pounds raw chicken bones and/or carcasses

1 whole chicken

4 to 6 chicken legs, thighs, or wings, optional

$\frac{1}{4}$ to $\frac{1}{2}$ cup apple cider vinegar

Purified water (enough to just cover the bones and meat)

2 to 4 carrots, scrubbed and roughly chopped

3 to 4 celery stalks, including leaves, roughly chopped

1 onion, cut into large chunks

1 tomato, cut into wedges, optional

1 to 2 garlic cloves

2 teaspoons black peppercorns

1 bunch parsley

In a large stockpot or slow cooker, add the bones, meat, vinegar, and enough water to cover everything by an inch. Cover the pot. Bring the water to a simmer over medium heat. Use a shallow spoon to carefully skim the film off the surface. If you're using a slow cooker, wait about 2 hours or until the water is warm before skimming, but in the meantime continue with the next step.

Add the carrots, celery, onion, tomato (if using), garlic, and peppercorns, reduce the heat to low, and cover. You want the broth to barely simmer. Skim occasionally during the first 2 hours. Cook for at least 6 hours or up to 8, adding water as needed to ensure the bones are always covered. During the last hour, add the parsley.

When the broth is done, remove the pot from the heat or turn off the cooker. Using tongs and/or a large slotted spoon, remove all the bones and meat (saving the chicken for another recipe). Pour the broth through a fine-mesh strainer and discard the solids.

Let the broth cool on the counter and refrigerate within 1 hour. You can skim off the fat again after the broth is chilled, if desired. When chilled, the broth should be very gelatinous—that collagen-based gelatin is a magic potion—*do not discard!* The broth will keep for 5 days in the refrigerator and 3 or more months in the freezer.

NOTES

If you're using a pressure cooker or Instant Pot, add all the ingredients and bring it up to full pressure (using the manufacturer's instructions). Reduce the heat to low, maintaining full pressure, and cook for 2 to 3 hours. Allow the pressure to naturally release.

You can also make this broth using rotisserie chicken carcasses and pieces.

Beef Bone Broth

PREP TIME: 15 min.

COOK TIME: 12 to 24 hrs.

YIELD: Varies depending on size of pot; these ingredients are sufficient for 1 gallon of broth

4 to 5 pounds pasture-raised beef bones, preferably marrow, joints, and knuckle bones

3 pounds meaty bones, such as oxtail, shank, or short ribs

$1/4$ to $1/2$ cup apple cider vinegar

Purified water (enough to just cover the bones and meat)

2 to 4 carrots, scrubbed and roughly chopped

2 celery stalks, including leaves, roughly chopped

1 onion, cut into large chunks

2 dried bay leaves

1 to 2 garlic cloves

1 tablespoon black peppercorns

In a large stockpot or slow cooker, add the bones, meat, vinegar, and enough water to cover everything by an inch. Cover the pot. Bring the water to a simmer over medium heat. Use a shallow spoon to carefully skim the film off the surface. If you're using a slow cooker, wait about 2 hours or until the water is warm before skimming, but in the meantime continue with the next step.

Add the carrots, celery, onion, bay leaves, garlic, and peppercorns, reduce the heat to low, and cover. You want the broth to barely simmer. Skim occasionally during the first 2 hours. Cook for at least 12 hours or up to 24, adding water as needed to ensure the bones are always covered.

When the broth is done, remove the pot from the heat or turn off the cooker. Using tongs and/or a large slotted spoon, remove all the bones and meat (saving the beef for another recipe). Pour the broth through a fine-mesh strainer and discard the solids.

Let cool on the counter and refrigerate within 1 hour. You can skim off the fat again after the broth is chilled, if desired. When chilled, the broth should be very gelatinous—that collagen-based gelatin is a magic potion—*do not discard!* The broth will keep for 5 days in the refrigerator and 3 or more months in your freezer.

NOTE

If you're using a pressure cooker or Instant Pot, add all the ingredients and bring it up to full pressure (using the manufacturer's instructions). Reduce the heat to low, maintaining full pressure, and cook for 2 to 3 hours. Allow the pressure to naturally release.

Fish Bone Broth

PREP TIME: 15 min.

COOK TIME: $1\frac{1}{4}$ hrs.

YIELD: Varies depending on size of pot; these ingredients are sufficient for 1 gallon of broth

5 to 7 pounds fish carcasses or heads from large non-oily fish, such as halibut, cod, sole, rockfish, turbot, or tilapia (see Notes)

2 tablespoons ghee

1 to 2 carrots, scrubbed and coarsely chopped

2 celery stalks, including leaves, coarsely chopped

2 onions, coarsely chopped

Purified water (enough just to cover the bones)

1 dried bay leaf

1 to 2 garlic cloves

2 teaspoons black peppercorns

1 tablespoon bouquet garni or small handful of fresh parsley with 4 to 5 stems of fresh thyme

Wash the fish and cut off the gills if present. Set aside.

In a large stockpot over low to medium-low heat, melt the ghee. Add the carrots, celery, and onions and cook, stirring occasionally, for about 20 minutes.

Add the fish and enough water to cover everything by an inch. Cover the pot. Bring the water to a simmer over medium heat. Use a shallow spoon to carefully skim the film off the surface. Add the bay leaf, garlic, peppercorns, and bouquet garni and reduce the heat to low. Cook at a bare simmer for about 50 minutes, uncovered or with the lid askew. Continue to skim the surface as needed.

When the broth is done, remove the pot from the heat. Using tongs and/or a large slotted spoon, remove all the bones. Pour the broth through a fine-mesh strainer and discard the solids.

Let cool on the counter and refrigerate within 1 hour. You can skim off the fat again after the broth is chilled, if desired. When chilled, the broth should be very gelatinous—that collagen-based gelatin is a magic potion—*do not discard!* The broth will keep for 5 days in the refrigerator and 3 or more months in your freezer.

NOTES

Non-oily fish is essential because the oils in fatty fish, such as salmon, can become rancid in extended cooking.

The cartilage in fish bones breaks down to gelatin very quickly, so it's best to cook this broth on the stovetop rather than in a pressure cooker or Instant Pot.

Sources Consulted

CHAPTER 1

Centre for Genetics Education. "An Introduction to DNA, RNA, Genes and Chromosomes." Updated September 2021. https://www.genetics.edu.au/publications-and-resources/facts-sheets/fact-sheet-1-an-introduction-to-dna-genes-and-chromosomes.

Koster, Maranke I. "Making an Epidermis." *Annals of the New York Academy of Sciences* vol. 1170: 7–10. doi:10.1111/j.1749-6632.2009.04363.x.

Lew, Virgilio L., and Teresa Tiffert. "On the Mechanism of Human Red Blood Cell Longevity: Roles of Calcium, the Sodium Pump, PIEZO1, and Gardos Channels." *Frontiers in Physiology* vol. 8: 977. doi:10.3389/fphys.2017.00977.

Minihane, Anne M., et al. "Low-Grade Inflammation, Diet Composition and Health: Current Research Evidence and Its Translation." *The British Journal of Nutrition* vol. 114, 7: 999–1012. doi:10.1017/S0007114515002093.

Paula Neto, Heitor A., et al. "Effects of Food Additives on Immune Cells as Contributors to Body Weight Gain and Immune-Mediated Metabolic Dysregulation." *Frontiers in Immunology* vol. 8: 1478. doi:10.3389/fimmu.2017.01478.

CHAPTER 2

Duffy, Eamon Y., et al. "Opportunities to Improve Cardiovascular Health in the New American Workplace." *American Journal of Preventive Cardiology* vol. 5: 100136. doi:10.1016/j.ajpc.2020.100136.

National Institute of General Medical Sciences. "Circadian Rhythms." Updated March 2022. https://www.nigms.nih.gov/education/fact-sheets/Pages/circadian-rhythms.aspx.

Ruhlman, Michael. *Grocery: The Buying and Selling of Food in America*. Abrams Press, 2017.

Sandoiu, Ana. "How Your Diet Can Keep Cells Healthy and Young." *Medical News Today*, August 22, 2018. https://www.medicalnewstoday.com/articles/322845.

Schaefer, Nathan K., et al. "An Ancestral Recombination Graph of Human, Neanderthal, and Denisovan Genomes." *Science Advances* vol. 7, 29. doi:10.1126/sciadv.abc0776.

Tuulari, Jetro J., et al. "Feeding Releases Endogenous Opioids in Humans." *Journal of Neuroscience* vol. 37, 34: 8284–8291. doi:10.1523/JNEUROSCI.0976-17.2017.

CHAPTER 3

Azaïs-Braesco, Véronique, et al. "A Review of Total & Added Sugar Intakes and Dietary Sources in Europe." *Nutrition Journal* vol. 16, 1: 6. doi:10.1186/s12937-016-0225-2.

Clegg, M. E., et al. "Soups Increase Satiety Through Delayed Gastric Emptying Yet Increased Glycaemic Response." *European Journal of Clinical Nutrition* vol. 67, 1: 8–11. doi:10.1038/ejcn.2012.152.

Harvard Health Publishing. "The Sweet Danger of Sugar." Updated January 2022. https://www.health.harvard.edu/heart-health/the-sweet-danger-of-sugar.

Kawai, Nobuhiro, et al. "The Sleep-Promoting and Hypothermic Effects of Glycine are Mediated by NMDA Receptors in the Suprachiasmatic Nucleus." *Neuropsychopharmacology* vol. 40, 6: 1405–1416. doi:10.1038/npp.2014.326.

Kim, Min-Hyun, and Hyeyoung Kim. "The Roles of Glutamine in the Intestine and Its Implication in Intestinal Diseases." *International Journal of Molecular Sciences* vol. 18, 5: 1051. doi:10.3390/ijms18051051.

Marcus, Jacqueline B. *Culinary Nutrition: The Science and Practice of Healthy Cooking*. Academic Press, 2013.

Marziali, M., et al. "Gluten-Free Diet: A New Strategy for Management of Painful Endometriosis Related Symptoms?" *Minerva Chirurgia* vol. 67, 6: 499–504.

Proksch, E., et al. "Oral Intake of Specific Bioactive Collagen Peptides Reduces Skin Wrinkles and Increases Dermal Matrix Synthesis." *Skin Pharmacology and Physiology* vol. 27, 3: 113–119. doi:10.1159/000355523.

———. "Oral Supplementation of Specific Collagen Peptides Has Beneficial Effects on Human Skin Physiology: A Double-Blind, Placebo-Controlled Study." *Skin Pharmacology and Physiology* vol. 27, 1: 47–55. doi:10.1159/000351376.

Rao, RadhaKrishna, and Geetha Samak. "Role of Glutamine in Protection of Intestinal Epithelial Tight Junctions." *Journal of Epithelial Biology & Pharmacology* vol. 5, suppl. 1-M7: 47–54. doi:10.2174/1875044301205010047.

Riebl, Shaun K., and Brenda M. Davy. "The Hydration Equation: Update on Water Balance and Cognitive Performance." *ACSM's Health & Fitness Journal* vol. 17, 6: 21–28. doi:10.1249/FIT.0b013e3182a9570f.

Wang, Bin, et al. "Glutamine and Intestinal Barrier Function." *Amino Acids* vol. 47, 10: 2143–2154. doi:10.1007/s00726-014-1773-4.

Wu, Guoyao, et al. "Proline and Hydroxyproline Metabolism: Implications for Animal and Human Nutrition." *Amino Acids* vol. 40, 4: 1053–1063. doi:10.1007/s00726-010 -0715-z.

Zhong, Zhi, et al. "L-Glycine: A Novel Anti-Inflammatory, Immunomodulatory, and Cytoprotective Agent." *Current Opinion in Clinical Nutrition and Metabolic Care* vol. 6, 2: 229–240. doi:10.1097/00075197-200303000-00013.

CHAPTER 4

Bacaro, Valeria, et al. "Sleep Duration and Obesity in Adulthood: An Updated Systematic Review and Meta-Analysis." *Obesity Research & Clinical Practice* vol. 14, 4: 301–309. doi:10.1016/j.orcp.2020.03.004.

Cappuccio, Francesco P., et al. "Sleep Duration Predicts Cardiovascular Outcomes: A Systematic Review and Meta-Analysis of Prospective Studies." *European Heart Journal* vol. 32, 12: 1484–1492. doi:10.1093/eurheartj/ehr007.

Cohut, Maria. "How Waste Gets 'Washed Out' of Our Brains During Sleep." *Medical News Today*, November 2, 2019. https://www.medicalnewstoday.com/articles /326896.

Dolezal, Brett A., et al. "Interrelationship Between Sleep and Exercise: A Systematic Review." *Advances in Preventive Medicine* vol. 2017: 1364387. doi:10.1155/2017/1364387.

Johns Hopkins Medicine. "The Science of Sleep." https://www.hopkinsmedicine.org/ health/wellness-and-prevention/the-science-of-sleep-understanding-what-happens -when-you-sleep.

Liu Y., et al. "Prevalence of Healthy Sleep Duration Among Adults—United States, 2014." *Morbidity and Mortality Weekly Report* vol. 65, 6: 137–141. doi:10.15585/mmwr .mm6506a1.

National Institute of General Medical Sciences. "Circadian Rhythms." Updated March 2022. https://www.nigms.nih.gov/education/fact-sheets/Pages/circadian-rhythms .aspx.

National Institute of Neurological Disorders and Stroke. "Brain Basics: Understanding Sleep." Updated April 2022. https://www.ninds.nih.gov/health-information/patient -caregiver-education/brain-basics-understanding-sleep.

Ochs-Balcom, Heather M., et al. "Short Sleep Is Associated with Low Bone Mineral Density and Osteoporosis in the Women's Health Initiative." *Journal of Bone and Mineral Research: The Official Journal of the American Society for Bone and Mineral Research* vol. 35, 2: 261–268. doi:10.1002/jbmr.3879.

Taheri, Shahrad, et al. "Short Sleep Duration Is Associated with Reduced Leptin, Elevated Ghrelin, and Increased Body Mass Index." *PLoS Medicine* vol. 1, 3: e62. doi:10.1371/journal.pmed.0010062.

Tähkämö, Leena et al. "Systematic Review of Light Exposure Impact on Human Circadian Rhythm." *Chronobiology International* vol. 36, 2: 151–170. doi:10.1080 /07420528.2018.1527773.

CHAPTER 5

American Psychological Association. "Working Out Boosts Brain Health." Updated March 2020. https://www.apa.org/topics/exercise-fitness/stress.

Colberg, Sheri R., and Carmine R. Grieco. "Exercise in the Treatment and Prevention of Diabetes." *Current Sports Medicine Reports* vol. 8, 4: 169–175. doi:10.1249 /JSR.0b013e3181ae0654.

Kraemer, William J., and Nicholas A. Ratamess. "Hormonal Responses and Adaptations to Resistance Exercise and Training." *Sports Medicine* vol. 35, 4: 339–361. doi:10.2165/00007256-200535040-00004.

Livingston, Gill, et al. "Dementia Prevention, Intervention, and Care." *Lancet* vol. 390, 10113: 2673–2734. doi:10.1016/S0140-6736(17)31363-6.

CHAPTER 6

Andre, Christophe. "Proper Breathing Brings Better Health." *Scientific American*, January 15, 2019. https://www.scientificamerican.com/article/proper-breathing-brings-better -health.

Arguinchona, Joseph H., and Prasanna Tadi. "Neuroanatomy, Reticular Activating System." *StatPearls*. https://www.ncbi.nlm.nih.gov/books/NBK549835.

Hamasaki, Hidetaka. "Effects of Diaphragmatic Breathing on Health: A Narrative Review." *Medicines* vol. 7, 10: 65. doi:10.3390/medicines7100065.

Joyner, Michael J., and Sarah E. Baker. "Take a Deep, Resisted, Breath." *Journal of the American Heart Association* vol. 10, 13: e022203. doi:10.1161/JAHA.121.022203.

Kaufman, Jason A. "Nature, Mind, and Medicine: A Model for Mind-Body Healing." *Explore* vol. 14, 4: 268–276. doi:10.1016/j.explore.2018.01.001.

Ranganathan, Vinoth K., et al. "From Mental Power to Muscle Power—Gaining Strength by Using the Mind." *Neuropsychologia* vol. 42, 7: 944–956. doi:10.1016/j .neuropsychologia.2003.11.018.

Walsh, Roger. "Lifestyle and Mental Health." *The American Psychologist* vol. 66, 7: 579–592. doi:10.1037/a0021769.

Wapner, Jessica. "Vision and Breathing May Be the Secrets to Surviving 2020." *Scientific American*, November 16, 2020. https://www.scientificamerican.com/article/vision -and-breathing-may-be-the-secrets-to-surviving-2020.

CHAPTER 7

Byrne, C. S., et al. "The Role of Short Chain Fatty Acids in Appetite Regulation and Energy Homeostasis." *International Journal of Obesity* vol. 39, 9: 1331–1338. doi:10.1038/ijo.2015.84.

DiNicolantonio, James J., and Sean C. Lucan. "Is Fructose Malabsorption a Cause of Irritable Bowel Syndrome?" *Medical Hypotheses* vol. 85, 3: 295–297. doi:10.1016/j .mehy.2015.05.019.

Fields, Helen. "The Gut: Where Bacteria and Immune System Meet." *John's Hopkins Medicine*, November 2015. https://www.hopkinsmedicine.org/research /advancements-in-research/fundamentals/in-depth/the-gut-where-bacteria-and -immune-system-meet.

Kim, M. H., and H. Kim. "The Roles of Glutamine in the Intestine and Its Implication in Intestinal Diseases." *International Journal of Molecular Sciences* vol. 18, 5: 1051. doi:10.3390/ijms18051051.

Kligler, Benjamin, and Sapna Chaudhary. "Peppermint Oil." *American Family Physician* vol. 75, 7: 1027–1030. https://www.aafp.org/pubs/afp/issues/2007/0401/p1027.html.

Marchesi, Julian R., et al. "The Gut Microbiota and Host Health: A New Clinical Frontier." *Gut* vol. 65, 2: 330–339. doi:10.1136/gutjnl-2015-309990.

Murciano-Brea, Julia, et al. "Gut Microbiota and Neuroplasticity." *Cells* vol. 10, 8: 2084. doi:10.3390/cells10082084.

National Institute of Diabetes and Digestion and Kidney Diseases. "Your Digestive System & How It Works." Updated December 2017. https://www.niddk.nih.gov /health-information/digestive-diseases/digestive-system-how-it-works.

Salem, Iman, et al. "The Gut Microbiome as a Major Regulator of the Gut-Skin Axis." *Frontiers in Microbiology* vol. 9: 1459. doi:10.3389/fmicb.2018.01459.

Vasim, Izzah, et al. "Intermittent Fasting and Metabolic Health." *Nutrients* vol. 14, 3: 631. doi:10.3390/nu14030631.

CHAPTER 8

Haslam, Danielle E., et al. "Beverage Consumption and Longitudinal Changes in Lipoprotein Concentrations and Incident Dyslipidemia in US Adults: The Framingham Heart Study." *Journal of the American Heart Association* vol. 9, 5: e014083. doi:10.1161/JAHA.119.014083.

Soliman, Ghada A. "Dietary Fiber, Atherosclerosis, and Cardiovascular Disease." *Nutrients* vol. 11, 5: 1155. doi:10.3390/nu11051155.

Turnbaugh, Peter J., et al. "A Core Gut Microbiome in Obese and Lean Twins." *Nature* vol. 457, 7228: 480–484. doi:10.1038/nature07540.

CHAPTER 9

Anand, Swadha, and Sharmila S. Mande. "Diet, Microbiota and Gut-Lung Connection." *Frontiers in Microbiology* vol. 9: 2147. doi:10.3389/fmicb.2018.02147.

Barrett, Deborah. "The Healing Powers of Sex." *Psychology Today*, November 6, 2011. https://www.psychologytoday.com/us/blog/paintracking/201111/the-healing-powers-sex.

Carr, Erikka L., et al. "Glutamine Uptake and Metabolism Are Coordinately Regulated by ERK/MAPK During T Lymphocyte Activation." *The Journal of Immunology* vol. 185, 2: 1037–1044. doi:10.4049/jimmunol.0903586.

Cleveland Clinic. "Thyroid Disease." Updated April 2020. https://my.clevelandclinic.org/health/diseases/8541-thyroid-disease.

———. "What Happens When Your Immune System Gets Stressed Out?" Updated March 2017. https://health.clevelandclinic.org/what-happens-when-your-immune-system-gets-stressed-out.

Franceschi, Claudio, et al. "Inflammaging: A New Immune-Metabolic Viewpoint for Age-Related Diseases." *Nature Reviews Endocrinology* vol. 14, 10: 576–590. doi:10.1038/s41574-018-0059-4.

Matenchuk, Brittany A., et al. "Sleep, Circadian Rhythm, and Gut Microbiota." *Sleep Medicine Reviews* vol. 53: 101340. doi:10.1016/j.smrv.2020.101340.

Mazaheri Nia, Leila, et al. "Effect of Zinc on Testosterone Levels and Sexual Function of Postmenopausal Women: A Randomized Controlled Trial." *Journal of Sex & Marital Therapy* vol. 47, 8: 804–813. doi:10.1080/0092623X.2021.1957732.

National Institute of Neurological Disorders and Stroke. "Brain Basics: Understanding Sleep." Updated April 2022. https://www.ninds.nih.gov/Disorders/patient-caregiver-education/understanding-sleep.

Parish, Sharon J., and Steven R. Hahn. "Hypoactive Sexual Desire Disorder: A Review of Epidemiology, Biopsychology, Diagnosis, and Treatment." *Sexual Medicine Reviews* vol. 4, 2: 103–120. doi:10.1016/j.sxmr.2015.11.009.

Suni, Eric. "How Sleep Deprivation Affects Your Heart." *Sleep Foundation*, April 1, 2022. https://www.sleepfoundation.org/sleep-deprivation/how-sleep-deprivation-affects-your-heart.

University of Cambridge. "Too Exhausted to Fight, Immune System May Harm the Body They Are Supposed to Protect." *ScienceDaily*, June 29, 2015. www.sciencedaily.com/releases/2015/06/150629110803.htm.

CHAPTER 10

American Chemical Society. "Scientists Say Vitamin C May Alleviate the Body's Response to Stress." *ScienceDaily*, August 23, 1999. www.sciencedaily.com /releases/1999/08/990823072615.htm.

Brookie, Kate L., et al. "Intake of Raw Fruits and Vegetables Is Associated with Better Mental Health than Intake of Processed Fruits and Vegetables." *Frontiers in Psychology* vol. 9: 487. doi:10.3389/fpsyg.2018.00487.

Caldwell, Emily. "Omega 3 Supplements Do Double Duty in Protecting Against Stress." *Ohio State News*, April 19, 2021. https://news.osu.edu/omega-3-supplements-do-double-duty-in-protecting-against -stress.

Chandrasekhar, K., et al. "A Prospective, Randomized Double-Blind, Placebo-Controlled Study of Safety and Efficacy of a High-Concentration Full-Spectrum Extract of Ashwagandha Root in Reducing Stress and Anxiety in Adults." *Indian Journal of Psychological Medicine* vol. 34, 3: 255–262. doi:10.4103/0253-7176.106022.

Cleveland Clinic. "What Happens When Your Immune System Gets Stressed Out?" Updated March 2017. https://health.clevelandclinic.org/what-happens-when-your -immune-system-gets-stressed-out.

Harvard Health Publishing. "Exercising to Relax." Updated July 2020. https://www .health.harvard.edu/staying-healthy/exercising-to-relax.

Hidese, Shinsuke, et al. "Effects of L-Theanine Administration on Stress-Related Symptoms and Cognitive Functions in Healthy Adults: A Randomized Controlled Trial." *Nutrients* vol. 11, 10: 2362. doi:10.3390/nu11102362.

Jennings, Kerri-Ann. "7 Reasons to Eat More Citrus Fruits." *HealthLine*, January 27, 2017. https://www.healthline.com/nutrition/citrus-fruit-benefits.

Lombardi, Lisa. "Why Fresh Berries Are the Most Healthy, Age-Fighting Foods Around." *Washington Post*. August 2, 2021.

Lovallo, William R., et al. "Caffeine Stimulation of Cortisol Secretion Across the Waking Hours in Relation to Caffeine Intake Levels." *Psychosomatic Medicine* vol. 67, 5: 734–739. doi:10.1097/01.psy.0000181270.20036.06.

Peters, Achim. "Why Do We Crave Sweets When We're Stressed?" *Scientific American*, February 27, 2019. https://www.scientificamerican.com/article/why-do-we-crave -sweets-when-were-stressed.

Pickering, Gisèle, et al. "Magnesium Status and Stress: The Vicious Circle Concept Revisited." *Nutrients* vol. 12, 12: 3672. doi:10.3390/nu12123672.

Steptoe, Andrew, et al. "The Effects of Tea on Psychophysiological Stress Responsivity and Post-Stress Recovery: A Randomised Double-Blind Trial." *Psychopharmacology* vol. 190, 1: 81–89. doi:10.1007/s00213-006-0573-2.

Terada, Yuki, et al. "Increased Anxiety-Like Behaviour Is an Early Symptom of Vitamin E Deficiency That Is Suppressed by Adrenalectomy in Rats." *British Journal of Nutrition* vol. 125, 11: 1310–1319. doi:10.1017/S0007114520001889.

CHAPTER 11

Choi, Franchesca D., et al. "Oral Collagen Supplementation: A Systematic Review of Dermatological Applications." *Journal of Drugs in Dermatology: JDD* vol. 18, 1: 9–16. https://pubmed.ncbi.nlm.nih.gov/30681787.

Environmental Working Group. "Guide to Sunscreens." https://www.ewg.org/sunscreen.

Holick, Michael F. "Shedding New Light on the Role of the Sunshine Vitamin D for Skin Health: The lncRNA-Skin Cancer Connection." *Experimental Dermatology* vol. 23, 6: 391–392. doi:10.1111/exd.12386.

Mead, M. Nathaniel. "Benefits of Sunlight: A Bright Spot for Human Health." *Environmental Health Perspectives* vol. 116, 4: A160–167. doi:10.1289/ehp.116-a160.

Paul, Cristiana, et al. "Significant Amounts of Functional Collagen Peptides Can Be Incorporated in the Diet While Maintaining Indispensable Amino Acid Balance." *Nutrients* vol. 11, 5: 1079. doi:10.3390/nu11051079.

Pullar, Juliet M., et al. "The Roles of Vitamin C in Skin Health." *Nutrients* vol. 9, 8: 866. doi:10.3390/nu9080866.

Salem, Iman, et al. "The Gut Microbiome as a Major Regulator of the Gut-Skin Axis." *Frontiers in Microbiology* vol. 9: 1459. doi:10.3389/fmicb.2018.01459.

Teo, Cheryl Wei Ling, et al. "Vitamin E in Atopic Dermatitis: From Preclinical to Clinical Studies." *Dermatology* vol. 237, 4: 553–564. doi:10.1159/000510653.

Umar, Meenakshi, et al. "Vitamin D and the Pathophysiology of Inflammatory Skin Diseases." *Skin Pharmacology and Physiology* vol. 31, 2: 74–86. doi:10.1159/000485132.

Žmitek, Katja, et al. "The Effect of Dietary Intake of Coenzyme Q10 on Skin Parameters and Condition: Results of a Randomised, Placebo-Controlled, Double-Blind Study." *BioFactors* vol. 43, 1: 132–140. doi:10.1002/biof.1316.

Index

turning back the clock through, 88–89
types of, 86–87
vibing, 87–90
exhaustion, 179–180, 181

Face Forward Principle, 242
Face Forward Recipes, 254–269
fairy dust foods, 62, 156–157
family, support from, 27–29
fasting, intermittent, 42, 56–58, 134–135,
    153–155
fat cells, sleep deprivation and, 71
fatigue, 179–180, 183, 184–185, 186, 191,
    193–195
fats, 46
fennel, 131, 172
fiber, 163–165, 199
Fish Bone Broth, 228–229, 275
FODMAP foods, 136
food
    automating, 51
    choosing of, 36–37
    80/20 program regarding, 60–63
    fairy dust, 62, 156–157
    as fillers, 38
    labels of, 48–50
    negative aspects of, 25
    overview of, 37
    purpose of, 38
    tastes-like-cardboard complex and, 39
    timeframes for, 78–79
    as transformation force blocker, 29–30
    transformation regarding, 37
fructose, 164–165
fruits
    benefits of, 197
    Berry Chia Parfait, 173
    Butternut-Apple Soup with Warming
        Spices, 230–231
    Chocolate Bark with Pistachios and
        Oranges, 210–211
    citrus, 43, 220–221
    Creamy Avocado Soup with Mango Salsa,
        256–257
    Cucumber-Melon Gazpacho, 146–147
    fiber within, 164–165
    Lemon Cheesecake Bars with Berry
        Topping, 268–269
    overview of, 47–48
    Strawberry-Almond Muffins, 237

GABA, 84
garlic, 43
gelatin, 41, 130
ginger, 131, 140, 200
glutamine, 130–131, 182
glutathione, 42
gluten, 36, 55, 158
glycine, 42, 75, 84
goal weight, 161–163
grains, 54, 136–137
grapefruit, 43
grey rock method, 28
gut, 40–41, 43–44, 52–56, 127–128, 135–137,
    181–182, 196, 245–246. *See also* digestion
gut-brain connection, 133–134

habits, development of, 16, 91–92
Halibut with Romesco Sauce recipe, 174–175
Hearty Beef Vegetable Soup recipe, 232–233
herbs, digestive, 131
high-fructose corn syrup, 137
hormones, 21, 90, 192–193, 194
hydration, 41, 59–60, 165, 251–252

illness, 72, 193–195
immune-boosting recipes, 200–211
immune system, 181
inflamm-aging, 188–189
inflammation, 148–149, 188–189
infusion cocktails, 251–252
intermittent fasting, 42, 56–58, 134–135,
    153–155
Italian Frittata with Sausage, Roasted Red
    Peppers, and Mushrooms recipe,
    206–207
Italian Vegetable Soup with Sausage and
    Fennel recipe, 172

je ne sais quoi, 6, 102
jicama, 132
joints, 41
journaling, 81

kimchi, 133
knowledge, power of, 14–16
kombucha, 132–133

labels, food, 48–50
Lemon Cheesecake Bars with Berry Topping
    recipe, 268–269

vegetables (*cont.*)

Broth with Mighty Greens, 168–169

Butternut-Apple Soup with Warming Spices, 230–231

Carrot-Ginger Soup, 142–143

Chicken Bone Broth, 272–273

Creamy Asparagus Soup, 167

Creamy Avocado Soup with Mango Salsa, 256–257

Creamy Broccoli Soup with Ginger, 201

cruciferous, 44

Cucumber-Melon Gazpacho, 146–147

for digestion, 132

Easy-Peasy Minted Pea Soup, 141

fibrous, 46–47

Fish Bone Broth, 275

as FODMAP foods, 136

for gut health, 44

Halibut with Romesco Sauce, 174–175

Hearty Beef Vegetable Soup, 232–233

Italian Frittata with Sausage, Roasted Red Peppers, and Mushrooms, 206–207

Italian Vegetable Soup with Sausage and Fennel, 172

Lemon Chicken, Asparagus, and Leeks with Pan Sauce, 176–177

Oyster Stew, 202–203

Pick-Me-Up Bone Broth, 200

Portuguese Sausage, Kale, and Potato Soup (Caldo Verde), 204

Quick-and-Easy Chicken Soup, 144–145

Salmon Chowder, 228–229

Salmon Tacos with Cabbage Slaw and Creamy Cilantro Dressing, 262–263

Sautéed Cod with Fresh Fennel, 148–149

Slow-Cooker Turkey and Sweet Potato Stew, 205

Spicy Seafood Soup (Caldo de Mariscos), 170–171

starchy, 47

stress and, 221–222

Sweet Potato Mash with Indian Spices, 208–209

Thai Sweet Potato Soup, 234–235

The Very Hungry Caterpillar (Carle), 217–218

vibing, 87–90

vision, 108–109

Vitamin A, 246

Vitamin C, 220–221, 223, 246, 249–250

Vitamin D, 85, 194, 198–199, 244, 250

Vitamin E, 223–224, 246, 250

wall squat, 94

water, 60, 165, 251–252. *See also* hydration

weight management

artificial sweeteners and, 160–161

carbohydrates and, 159

challenges of, 151

dairy and, 159

80/20 program and, 156–157

emotional-eating management and, 155–156

fiber and, 163–165

gluten and, 158

goal weight and, 161–163

intermittent fasting and, 153–154

sleep deprivation and, 71

slim-gestion and, 152–153

snacks and, 159

sugar and, 160

through exercise, 89

viewpoints regarding, 150–151

water and, 165

wellness, 25, 70, 150, 243

yogurt, 133

zinc, 198, 251

ABOUT THE AUTHOR

Kellyann Petrucci, MS, ND, is a board-certified naturopathic physician, a certified nutrition consultant, and the author of five books, including the *New York Times* bestseller *Dr. Kellyann's Bone Broth Diet* and *The 10-Day Belly Slimdown*. A concierge doctor for celebrities in New York and Los Angeles, Dr. Kellyann has been a host for Public Television specials and has been featured on *Dr. Oz, The Doctors, Good Morning America,* and *Today.*